Sleep Medicine: Current Challenges and its Future

Editor

BARBARA GNIDOVEC STRAŽIŠAR

SLEEP MEDICINE CLINICS

www.sleep.theclinics.com

Consulting Editor
TEOFILO LEE-CHIONG Jr

September 2021 • Volume 16 • Number 3

ELSEVIER

1600 John F. Kennedy Boulevard • Suite 1800 • Philadelphia, Pennsylvania, 19103-2899

http://www.theclinics.com

SLEEP MEDICINE CLINICS Volume 16, Number 3
September 2021, ISSN 1556-407X, ISBN-13: 978-0-323-89730-3

Editor: Joanna Collett
Developmental Editor: Axell Ivan Jade M. Purificacion

Sleep Medicine Clinics (ISSN 1556-407X) is published quarterly by Elsevier Inc., 360 Park Avenue South, New York, NY 10010-1710. Months of issue are March, June, September and December. Business and Editorial Offices: 1600 John F. Kennedy Blvd., Ste. 1800, Philadelphia, PA 19103-2899. Customer Service Office: 3251 Riverport Lane, Maryland Heights, MO 63043. Periodicals postage paid at New York, NY and additional mailing offices. Subscription prices are $225.00 per year (US individuals), $100.00 (US and Canadian students), $625.00 (US institutions), $272.00 (Canadian individuals), $252.00 (international individuals), $135.00 (International students), $656.00 (Canadian and International institutions). Foreign air speed delivery is included in all *Clinics* subscription prices. All prices are subject to change without notice. **POSTMASTER:** Send change of address to *Sleep Medicine Clinics*, Elsevier Health Sciences Division, Subscription Customer Service, 3251 Riverport Lane, Maryland Heights, MO 63043. Customer Service: **Tel: 1-800-654-2452 (U.S. and Canada); 314-447-8871 (outside U.S. and Canada). Fax: 314-447-8029. E-mail: journalscustomerservice-usa@elsevier.com (for print support); journalsonline-support-usa@elsevier.com (for online support).**

Reprints. For copies of 100 or more of articles in this publication, please contact the Commercial Reprints Department, Elsevier Inc., 360 Park Avenue South, New York, NY 10010-1710. Tel.: 212-633-3874; Fax: 212-633-3820; E-mail: reprints@elsevier.com.

Sleep Medicine Clinics is covered in *MEDLINE/PubMed (Index Medicus)*.

Printed in the United States of America.

SLEEP MEDICINE CLINICS

FORTHCOMING ISSUES

December 2021
Measuring Sleep
Erna Sif Arnardóttir, *Editor*

March 2022
Causes of Sleep Complaints
Keith Aguilera and Agnes Remulla, *Editors*

RECENT ISSUES

June 2021
Movement Disorders in Sleep
Diego Garcia-Borreguero, *Editor*

March 2021
Piecing Together the Puzzle of Adherence in Sleep Medicine
Jessie P. Bakker, *Editor*

December 2020
Noninvasive Ventilation
Lisa F. Wolfe and Amen Sergew, *Editors*

SERIES OF RELATED INTEREST

Clinics in Chest Medicine
Available at: https://www.chestmed.theclinics.com/

THE CLINICS ARE AVAILABLE ONLINE!
Access your subscription at:
www.theclinics.com

Contributors

CONSULTING EDITOR

TEOFILO LEE-CHIONG Jr, MD
Professor of Medicine, National Jewish Health,
University of Colorado Denver, Denver,
Colorado; Chief Medical Liaison, Philips
Respironics, Pennsylvania

EDITOR

BARBARA GNIDOVEC STRAŽIŠAR, MD, PhD
President of the Slovenian Sleep Society, Head
of Paediatric Department and Director of
Centre for Paediatric Sleep Disorders, Former
Head of Executive Committee Assembly of
National Sleep Society (ANSS), Associate
Professor, General Hospital Celje and College
of Nursing in Celje, Celje, Slovenia

AUTHORS

ERNA SIF ARNARDOTTIR, PhD
Reykjavik University Sleep Institute, School of
Technology, Reykjavik University, Internal
Medicine Services, Landspitali University
Hospital, Reykjavik, Iceland

MIKHAIL BOCHKAREV, MD, PhD
Senior Researcher, Sleep Laboratory,
Research Department for Hypertension,
Almazov National Medical Research Centre, St
Petersburg, Russia

INGO FIETZE, MD, PhD
Professor, Charité Universitätsmedizin Berlin,
Interdisciplinary Sleep Medicine Center, Berlin,
Germany

MARTIN GLOS, PhD
Charité Universitätsmedizin Berlin,
Interdisciplinary Sleep Medicine Center, Berlin,
Germany

LUDGER GROTE, MD, PhD
Center for Sleep and Vigilance Disorders,
Sahlgrenska Academy, University of
Gothenburg, Sleep Disorders Center,
Respiratory Department, Sahlgrenska
University Hospital, Gothenburg, Sweden

JAN HEDNER, MD, PhD
Center for Sleep and Vigilance Disorders,
Sahlgrenska Academy, University of
Gothenburg, Sleep Disorders Center,
Respiratory Department, Sahlgrenska
University Hospital, Gothenburg, Sweden

ANNA SIGRIDUR ISLIND, PhD
Reykjavik University Sleep Institute, School of
Technology, Reykjavik University, Department
of Computer Science, Reykjavik University,
Reykjavik, Iceland

SAMSON G. KHACHATRYAN, MD, PhD
Chairman, Neurologist, Somnologist (ESRS cert.), Clinic Director, Department of Neurology and Neurosurgery, National Institute of Health, Ministry of Health, Sleep and Movement Disorders Center, Somnus Neurology Clinic, Yerevan, Armenia

LYUDMILA KOROSTOVTSEVA, MD, PhD
Senior Researcher, Sleep Laboratory, Research Department for Hypertension, Associate Professor, Department for Cardiology, Almazov National Medical Research Centre, St Petersburg, Russia

WALTER T. McNICHOLAS, MD
Professor, School of Medicine, University College Dublin, Department of Respiratory and Sleep Medicine, St. Vincent's Hospital Group, Consultants' Clinic, St Vincent's Private Hospital, Elm Park, Dublin, Ireland

CARLOTTA MUTTI, MD
Sleep Disorders Center, Department of Medicine and Surgery, Neurology Unit, University of Parma, Parma, Italy

MARÍA ÓSKARSDÓTTIR, PhD
Reykjavik University Sleep Institute, School of Technology, Reykjavik University, Department of Computer Science, Reykjavik University, Reykjavik, Iceland

LIBORIO PARRINO, MD, PhD
Sleep Disorders Center, Department of Medicine and Surgery, Neurology Unit, University of Parma, Parma, Italy

THOMAS PENZEL, PhD
Professor, Charité Universitätsmedizin Berlin, Interdisciplinary Sleep Medicine Center, Berlin, Germany

DIRK PEVERNAGIE, MD, PhD
Department of Respiratory Medicine, Ghent University Hospital, Department of Internal Medicine and Paediatrics, Faculty of Medicine and Health Sciences, Ghent University, Gent, Belgium

FRANCESCO RAUSA, MD
Sleep Disorders Center, Department of Medicine and Surgery, Neurology Unit, University of Parma, Parma, Italy

BARBARA GNIDOVEC STRAŽIŠAR, MD, PhD
President of the Slovenian Sleep Society, Head of Paediatric Department and Director of Centre for Paediatric Sleep Disorders, Former Head of Executive Committee Assembly of National Sleep Society (ANSS), Associate Professor, General Hospital Celje and College of Nursing in Celje, Celje, Slovenia

LEA STRAŽIŠAR
Student, CMS - Center for Sleep Disorders, Ljubljana, Slovenia

YURII SVIRYAEV, MD, PhD
Head, Sleep Laboratory, Research Department for Hypertension, World-Class Research Centre for Personalized Medicine, Almazov National Medical Research Centre, St Petersburg, Russia

JENNY THEORELL-HAGLÖW, RN, PhD
Department of Medical Sciences, Respiratory, Allergy and Sleep Research, Uppsala University, The Sleep Apnea Center, Respiratory Department, Uppsala University Hospital, Uppsala, Sweden

MARTIN ULANDER, MD, PhD
Department of Clinical Neurophysiology, Linköping University Hospital, Department of Biomedical and Clinical Sciences, Faculty of Medicine, Linköping University, Linköping, Sweden

JOHAN VERBRAECKEN, MD, PhD
Department of Pulmonary Medicine and Multidisciplinary Sleep Disorders Centre, Antwerp University Hospital, University of Antwerp, Edegem, Antwerp, Belgium

Contents

The worldwide COVID-19 pandemic has affected the operation of health care systems. The direct impact of obstructive sleep apnea (OSA) on COVID-19 infection outcome remains to be elucidated. However, the coincidence of common risk factors for OSA and severe COVID-19 suggests that patients with OSA receiving positive airway pressure therapy may have an advantage relative to those untreated when confronted with a COVID-19 infection. The ongoing COVID-19 pandemic has led to a substantial reduction of sleep medicine services, and the long-term consequences may be considerable. New strategies for the management of sleep disorders are needed to overcome the current underdiagnosis and delay of treatment.

Interest in telemedicine has increased exponentially. There is a growing body of published evidence on the use of telemedicine for patients using continuous positive airway pressure. Telemedicine-ready devices can support the transmission on use time, apnea–hypopnea index, and leakage. This approach enables early activation of troubleshooting. Automated, personalized feedback for patients and patient access to their own data provide unprecedented opportunities for integrating comanagement approaches, multiactor interactions, and patient empowerment. Telemedicine is likely cost effective, but requires better evidence. Notwithstanding barriers for implementation that remain, telemedicine has to be embraced, leaving the physician and patient to accept it or not.

This article provides an overview of the current use, limitations, and future directions of the variety of subjective and objective sleep assessments available. This article argues for various ways and sources of collecting, combining, and using data to enlighten clinical practice and the sleep research of the future. It highlights the prospects of digital management platforms to store and present the data, and the importance of codesign when developing such platforms and other new instruments. It also discusses the abundance of opportunities that data science and machine learning open for the analysis of data.

Sleep disorders are categorized in line with traditional taxonomy. This conventional approach allows adequate management of many patients. Failure of treatment, however, may be due to nonspecificity of symptoms, coincidental association between symptoms and pathophysiological endotype, as well as co-occurrence of different pathologic mechanisms affecting sleep. Complex phenotypes often do not respond well to standard therapeutic interventions. In these cases, the clinical workup should aim at identifying treatable traits that will likely improve under targeted therapy. The challenge for sleep medicine is to further develop this innovative approach that is driven by the principles of systems medicine.

New trends in sleep medicine make use of the increased computational power of digital transformation. A current trend toward fewer sensors on the body of the sleeper and to more data processing from derived signals is observed. Telemedicine technologies are used for data transmission and for better patient management in terms of diagnosis and in terms of treatment of chronic conditions.

Sleep is essential for healthy being and healthy functioning of human body as a whole, as well as each organ and system. Sleep disorders, such as sleep-disordered breathing, insomnia, sleep fragmentation, and sleep deprivation are associated with the deterioration in human body functioning and increased cardiovascular risks. However, owing to the complex regulation and heterogeneous state sleep per se can be associated with cardiovascular dysfunction in susceptible subjects. The understanding of sleep as a multidimensional concept is important for better prevention and treatment of cardiovascular diseases.

Sleep is a complex brain state with fundamental relevance for cognitive functions, synaptic plasticity, brain resilience, and autonomic balance. Sleep pathologies may interfere with cerebral circuit organization, leading to negative consequences and favoring the development of neurologic disorders. Conversely, the latter can interfere with sleep functions. Accordingly, assessment of sleep quality is always recommended in the diagnosis of patients with neurologic disorders and during neurorehabilitation programs. This review investigates the complex interplay between sleep and brain pathologies, focusing on diseases in which the association with sleep disturbances is commonly overlooked and whereby major benefits may derive from their proper management.

Insomnia is an important but widely ignored health problem in modern society. Despite unequivocal evidence on its large prevalence, health and social impacts, comorbidities, and various pharmacologic and nonpharmacologic (behavioral and device-based) approaches, its effective management is still difficult and often incomplete. This article discusses the role of insomnia in modern societies, newer complicating factors, and its overall social and public health burden. Acute insomnia and sleep difficulties during pandemic and confinement are reviewed. The article also focuses on newer developments accumulating in the field of insomnia and possible future trends.

Daylight Saving Time: Pros and Cons

Barbara Gnidovec Stražišar and Lea Stražišar

The original rationale for the adoption of daylight saving time (DST) was to conserve energy; however, the effects of DST on energy consumption are questionable or negligible. Conversely, there is substantial evidence that DST transitions have the cumulative effect on sleep deprivation with its adverse health effects. In light of current evidence, the European Commission in 2018 decided that biannual clock change in Europe would be abolished. Current indirect evidence supports the adoption of perennial standard time, which aligns best with the human circadian system and has the potential to produce benefits for public health and safety.

Sleepiness Behind the Wheel and the Implementation of European Driving Regulations

Walter T. McNicholas

Sleep disturbance and sleepiness are established risk factors for driving accidents and obstructive sleep apnea (OSA) is the most prevalent medical disorder associated with excessive daytime sleepiness. Because effective treatment of OSA reduces accident risk, several jurisdictions have implemented regulations concerning the ability of patients with OSA to drive, unless effectively treated. This review provides a practical guide for clinicians who may be requested to certify a patient with OSA as fit to drive regarding the scope of the problem, the role of questionnaires and driving simulators to evaluate sleepiness, and the benefit of treatment on accident risk.

Preface
Sleep Medicine: A Wise Investment

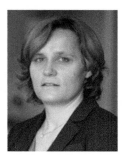

Barbara Gnidovec Stražišar, MD, PhD
Editor

Sleep medicine is a young, interdisciplinary medical field that over the past decades slowly and persistently paved its way through diverse health care systems in different parts of the world. There is no doubt that good and sufficient sleep is essential for health and well-being. However, with growing demands to the health care systems brought by aging of the population and special circumstances, like the current COVID-19 pandemic, there is justified fear that diagnosing and treating sleep disorders might in the future face less affection from health care decison makers.

Conventional in-lab sleep diagnostics is often laborious and expensive; therefore, future trends in sleep medicine should be oriented to the evaluation of sleep-disordered patients in a more naturalistic home environment with monitoring devices that are less obtrusive, more accessible, and yet still reliable. Various types of ambulatory recordings have already been introduced in the clinical practice, and these should form the basis for future development of various ambulatory treatment interventions.

This special issue is addressing these challenges and offers possible solutions with new trends and evolving technology in sleep medicine. These will allow better accessibility for the detection and treatment of sleep disorders in different populations and different circumstances.

The COVID-19 pandemic reduced sleep medicine services in many parts of the world and at the same time accelerated the use of telemedicine in the field of sleep medicine, especially in the management of sleep-disordered breathing. Telemedicine is an emerging field that has currently recieved widespread acceptance among diverse medical specialities and offers also tremendous possibilities in sleep medicine for diagnosing, treatment, and long-term follow-up of sleep-disordered patients. There is, however, an obvious need for improved subjective and objective measurements of sleep. New trends in sleep medicine make use of digital management platforms for storing and presenting the data, while data science with machine learning offers new analysis of the sleep data. This can facilitate the discovery of new important patterns and novel insight in sleep data. The methodology can also help in identifying certain clinical trends for more targeted treatment and thus challenge the conventional approach to the management of sleep disorders that is often insufficient in complex phenotypes. With growing knowledge in sleep medicine, there is a parallel growth of technical solutions for less-obtrusive sensors for sleep monitoring and at the same time more data processing for improving patient management strategies.

Sleep Med Clin 16 (2021) xi–xii
https://doi.org/10.1016/j.jsmc.2021.06.001
1556-407X/21/© 2021 Published by Elsevier Inc.

These are essential since sleep is important for every aspect of our health. Sleep disorders are associated with deterioration in human body functioning with increased cardiovascular risks, which can lead to negative consequences favoring the development of neurologic disorders. More prevalent sleep disorders, such as insomnia, are associated also with great economic and social burden, where direct and indirect costs far outweigh the burden of the treatment. Thus, in the future, we must be more aware also of important aspects of sleep medicine for the general public well-being, such as the importance of sleep and sleep-disordered breathing for traffic regulation and the influence of seasonal changing of the clock to human sleep.

Barbara Gnidovec Stražišar, MD, PhD
General Hospital Celje
College of Nursing in Celje
Mariborska cesta 7
3000 Celje, Slovenia

E-mail address:
barbara.gnidovec-strazisar@sb-celje.si

Prolonged Effects of the COVID-19 Pandemic on Sleep Medicine Services— Longitudinal Data from the Swedish Sleep Apnea Registry

Ludger Grote, MD, PhD[a,b,*], Jenny Theorell-Haglöw, RN, PhD[c,d], Martin Ulander, MD, PhD[e,f], Jan Hedner, MD, PhD[a,b]

KEYWORDS

- CPAP • Sleep test • Diagnosis • Mandibular advancement device • Polysomnography
- SARS-COV2 • Obstructive sleep apnea • Delivery of health care

KEY POINTS

- The ongoing COVID-19 pandemic has led to a substantial reduction of sleep medicine services, and the long-term consequences may be considerable.
- Recent data from the National Swedish Sleep Apnea Registry suggested important overall reduction of sleep diagnostic procedures and obstructive sleep apnea (OSA) treatment starts.
- The patients with OSA receiving positive airway pressure therapy may have an advantage relative to those untreated when confronted with a COVID-19 infection.
- New strategies for the management of sleep disorders are needed to overcome the current underdiagnosis and delay of treatment, including patients with OSA who potentially may be on high risk for severe COVID-19.
- Novel clinical routines such as the use of telemedicine may facilitate the recovery of sleep medicine services.

INTRODUCTION

The COVID-19 pandemic has affected the operation of health care systems. Resources have been shifted from elective care to acute management of severely ill patients affected by life-threatening infections with SARS-COV2. Experiences from virus outbreaks in China, Europe, and America as well as the announcement of a COVID-19 pandemic by the World Health Organization in March 2020 have sparked extensive and wide-ranging organizational changes in the health care system.

According to current recommendations from several expert organizations, sleep medicine centers are advised to reduce in-laboratory (in-lab) activities such as diagnostic polysomnography or positive airway pressure (PAP) titration, to provide

[a] Center for Sleep and Vigilance Disorders, Sahlgrenska Academy, University of Gothenburg, Medicinaregatan 8B, Box 421, 40530 Gothenburg, Sweden; [b] Respiratory Department, Sleep Disorders Center, Sahlgrenska University Hospital, 41345 Gothenburg, Sweden; [c] Department of Medical Sciences, Respiratory, Allergy and Sleep Research, Uppsala University, Akademiska sjukhuset ing 40, 75185 Uppsala, Sweden; [d] Respiratory Department, The Sleep Apnea Center, Uppsala University Hospital, 75185 Uppsala, Sweden; [e] Department of Clinical Neurophysiology, Linköping University Hospital, 58185 Linköping, Sweden; [f] Department of Biomedical and Clinical Sciences, Faculty of Medicine, Linköping University, 58185 Linköping, Sweden
* Corresponding author. Center for Sleep and Vigilance Disorders, Sahlgrenska Academy, University of Gothenburg, Medicinaregatan 8B, Box 421, 40530 Gothenburg, Sweden.
E-mail address: ludger.grote@lungall.gu.se

Sleep Med Clin 16 (2021) 409–416
https://doi.org/10.1016/j.jsmc.2021.05.008
1556-407X/21/© 2021 The Authors. Published by Elsevier Inc.

medical care by distance contact over phone or video calls, and to use telemedicine solutions for the diagnosis and treatment of sleep-disordered breathing.[1–6]

Treatment of sleep-disordered breathing with PAP or noninvasive ventilation during a COVID-19 infection has sparked a lively discussion on the pros and cons of the therapy.[7,8] Noninvasive ventilation has been suggested to cause increased risk for infection particularly among surrounding family members, care givers, or other patients due to aerosol dispersion via the vented mask.[9] An individual decision may therefore be needed not only in terms of continuation of treatment but also with respect to implementation of various countermeasures (nonvented masks with filters, self-isolation, opening of windows, protection of care givers and other patients).[2–4]

In this review the authors highlight important aspects for a possible association between sleep-disordered breathing, in particular OSA, and COVID-19 and the influence of the COVID-19 pandemic on sleep medicine services. They present the first quantitative analysis on the change of OSA management during 2020 based on data from a Swedish national registry.

SLEEP-DISORDERED BREATHING AS A RISK FACTOR FOR COVID-19 INFECTIONS AND WORSE OUTCOME

OSA is a prevalent and chronic disease,[10] and many patients with OSA suffer from cardiometabolic comorbidities.[11] Interestingly, risk factors for sleep apnea (male gender, higher age, obesity, hypertension, ischemic heart disease, arrhythmia, and diabetes mellitus) correspond to the identified risk factors for worse outcome following severe COVID-19 infections.[12] The direct impact of sleep apnea on COVID-19 infection outcome remains to be elucidated, but the coincidence of those risk factors suggests that patients with OSA may face an overall increased risk for severe COVID-19 infections and that they may benefit from ongoing therapy if confronted with a COVID-19 infection.[13]

Indeed, several retrospective studies support this hypothesis. A register-based study from Korea including 36,350 patients with chronic respiratory disease and 85,675 controls identified OSA as a risk factor for COVID-19 infection but not for mortality.[14] In addition, a Finish study performed in 445 individuals diagnosed with COVID-19 identified an increased risk for hospitalization in those with previously diagnosed OSA (n = 38).[13] Fifty percent of the individuals were hospitalized due to severe COVID-19, which corresponded to an almost 3-fold risk increase (adjusted odds ratio [OR] 2.98, $P = .0048$). In

the same paper, the investigators performed a meta-analysis of all studies published so far and identified OSA as a risk factor in the models adjusted for age and sex (OR 2.36, 95% confidence interval [CI] 1.14–4.95), but the increased risk was no longer significant after control for body mass index (OR 1.55, 95% CI 0.88–2.72). Further, a local US-based registry study identified 6.3% patients with OSA among 9405 patients with COVID-19 compared with a 0.3% OSA prevalence in the reference material.[15] For patients with OSA, the adjusted OR was 1.65 (95% CI 1.36–2.02) for COVID-19–related hospitalization and 1.98 (95% CI 1.63–2.37) for COVID-19–related respiratory failure when compared with non-OSA controls.[15] In contrast, another study from a large hospital-based registry identified no association between an OSA diagnosis and COVID-19–related outcome.[16]

Further evidence comes from a recent prospective, questionnaire-based study investigating 320 subjects referred to hospital with a COVID-19 infection.[17] An increased risk for worse clinical outcome in terms of need for intensive care unit treatment, oxygen supply, or delayed recovery over time was observed in subjects with a history of loud snoring and an elevated risk of OSA according to the Berlin questionnaire score. Although OSA was not assessed by means of an objective sleep test and only a subgroup (61%) had polymerase chain reaction (PCR)-verified COVID-19, these data suggest that OSA-related factors may play a role in the development of a complicated COVID-19 infection.[17]

In summary, several studies have identified OSA as a potential independent risk factor for severe COVID-19 infections. The exact effect size is difficult to determine due to the high prevalence of comorbidities, in particular obesity, metabolic, and cardiovascular disease. Further prospective studies may benefit from objective assessment of OSA intensity and nocturnal hypoxia as well as a rigorous mapping of comorbidities in both cases and controls.

INFLUENCE OF THE COVID-19 PANDEMIC ON SLEEP MEDICINE SERVICES
Existing Evidence

Several studies have explored the changes of sleep medicine services worldwide. One of the first studies, performed in Europe, explored the change in clinical practice observed in the European Sleep Apnea Database network.[18] The impact of the COVID-19 pandemic on the management of patients with OSA was assessed by a questionnaire answered by 40 sleep centers in 15 European countries at the time of the first lockdown (March/April 2020). Sleep medicine services were dramatically reduced, and staffing levels were decreased to 25%/19% for physicians/nurses and technicians, respectively, when compared with prepandemic baseline. However, a substantial difference in staffing levels between European regions was identified (**Fig. 1**). Sleep-disordered breathing diagnosis by in-lab polysomnography/home sleep testing was reduced from 93%/88% before COVID-19 to 20%/33%, respectively (**Fig. 2**). In-lab PAP titration was stopped at 72% of sleep centers, whereas it was still ongoing in 18% (**Fig. 3**). Follow-up by phone or video calls were performed by 75% of the centers but only 25% allowed for a physical meeting with the patient. At that time of the pandemic, telemedicine-based service had been initiated at some clinics and was performed in only one-third of centers. The data suggest a substantial close-down of sleep medicine services around Europe following the first wave of the COVID-19 pandemic. New strategies such as telemedicine-based practice seemed to be insufficiently exploited.

These results are further supported by several studies investigating the change of sleep medicine practice during the pandemic by means of questionnaires (**Table 1**). The most comprehensive study so far included 297 American Academy of Sleep Medicine–associated sleep centers located predominantly in the United States and in Canada.[19] The lockdown of activities was even more pronounced with greater than 90% reduction of in-lab diagnostic and therapeutic procedures. Mitigation strategies were applied with less

extensive mask fitting procedures, PCR testing before visits, or a change to home sleep testing.[1,3] The picture of a worldwide reduction of activities is further completed by a study from China.[20] In 56 centers spread out over the country, sleep medicine services were reduced with almost 90% during the first wave of the pandemic. Subsequently, the activities recovered during summer 2020 to an approximately 50% level when compared with prepandemic baseline. Further local, regional, and national surveys may have been performed without publication in international journals, but such estimates are usually based on qualitative point assessments. There is an obvious lack of longitudinal and quantitative patient data following the dynamics of the pandemic, which prompted a specific analysis of data from the national Swedish Sleep Apnea Registry (SESAR).

Novel Quantitative Data from the Swedish Sleep Apnea Registry

SESAR is one out of the 100 national quality registries in Sweden and was started in 2010. SESAR collects patient data from sleep centers involved in the different aspects of sleep apnea management: diagnosis, treatment, and follow-up. In 2019, data from 23,636 unselected patient visits have been manually entered by 35 sleep centers across Sweden.[22] The data were obtained at the end of the diagnostic procedure and at the start of the 2 main treatment modalities—PAP and mandibular advancement devices (MAD). A total of 7623 follow-up visits were reported mainly related to PAP therapy (n = 6625). The overall

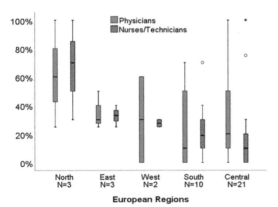

Fig. 1. Staffing in sleep medicine services (in %) during the COVID-19 pandemic in comparison to regular service (corresponding to 100%) in various European regions. (Data reported in Grote L, McNicholas WT, Hedner J; ESADA collaborators. Sleep apnoea management in Europe during the COVID-19 pandemic: data from the European Sleep Apnoea Database (ESADA). Eur Respir J. 2020 Jun 18;55(6):2001323.)

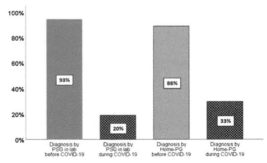

Fig. 2. Changes in the routine of diagnostic procedures during the COVID-19 pandemic demonstrating the marked reduction in both in-laboratory polysomnography (PSG) and ambulatory cardiorespiratory polygraphy (PG). Data are presented as percentage of centers reporting PSG or home-PG use. (Data reported in Grote L, McNicholas WT, Hedner J; ESADA collaborators. Sleep apnoea management in Europe during the COVID-19 pandemic: data from the European Sleep Apnoea Database (ESADA). Eur Respir J. 2020 Jun 18;55(6):2001323.)

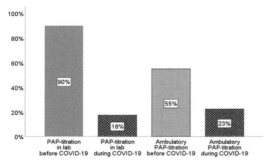

Fig. 3. Changes in the routine of PAP treatment initiation for patients with sleep apnea during the COVID-19 pandemic demonstrating the marked reduction in both in-laboratory and ambulatory initiation. Data are presented as percentage of centers reporting in laboratory or ambulatory PAP titration. (Data reported in Grote L, McNicholas WT, Hedner J; ESADA collaborators. Sleep apnoea management in Europe during the COVID-19 pandemic: data from the European Sleep Apnoea Database (ESADA). Eur Respir J. 2020 Jun 18;55(6):2001323.)

national coverage of sleep apnea services has been calculated to exceed 60% for diagnostic procedures and PAP starts and approximately 20% for MAD. Clinically relevant results of the registry are publicly available on the registry webpage (www.sesar.se/statistik), which illustrates between-centre comparisons of patient characteristics, waiting times, and treatment outcomes (eg, adherence to PAP, mandibular advancement for MAD, proportion of initiated weight reduction therapy in obese patients with OSA).

For the purpose of the current analysis the authors compiled data on patient recruitment during the period March to December 2020 and compared with results from an identical time window of the 2 preceding years (March–December 2018/2019). The mean number of patients registered each month during 2018/19 was calculated and used as a baseline to calculate and plot the change from baseline during year 2020.

Although there were fewer restrictions related to COVID-19 in the Swedish society, the access to routine health service was significantly reduced mainly in hospitals. As most of the sleep medicine services are centralized at the regional hospitals, access to sleep tests or PAP treatment starts was substantially reduced in those units. In addition, many patients did not show up for scheduled visits due to a perceived increased risk for virus infection. Also, people with common cold symptoms, which are prevalent in Sweden during autumn and winter, were instructed to self-quarantine.

Data from the SESAR registry show a sharp decline in sleep apnea services throughout the

entire time window during 2020 (**Fig. 4**). Compared with baseline from 2018/2019, sleep diagnostic procedures and PAP titrations declined by 50% before the summer period 2020. After summer, when the virus spreading in the Swedish society was relatively low, some activities recovered very slowly. Subsequently, it was mainly home titration of PAP treatment that fully recovered despite a second wave of the pandemic. Even higher infection rates during November and December 2020 did not change the recovery of PAP titrations. On the contrary, the treatment start of oral devices (MAD) declined even during the second half of the year without any signs of recovery. Further detailed analysis of patient characteristics may be warranted to fully understand the potential selection and prioritization process at the different sleep centers reporting to the SESAR registry.

Reopening of Sleep Medicine Services During the Pandemic

The data listed earlier clearly demonstrate a large impact of the COVID-19 pandemic on sleep medicine services in many areas of the world. Several important findings need to be pointed out. First, sleep medicine service has been substantially reduced by 50% to 90% during the first 10 to 12 months of the global COVID-19 pandemic. Second, in-house procedures, including supervised polysomnography or in-lab PAP titrations, are performed in small scale or not at all or only in a very limited fashion in highly selected patient groups. This change in practice may not fully apply to those countries where home sleep testing and automated PAP titration have been performed even before the pandemic. Third, initiation of PAP treatment of sleep-disordered breathing is significantly reduced and may have recovered at least in some countries. This may in part be the results of a medical prioritization in sleep medicine centers. Fourth, the full potential of mitigation strategies, including telemedicine approaches for diagnosis, treatment initiation, or follow-up of patients with sleep-disordered breathing, has not been studied in more detail. It is anticipated that the use of these new technologies may be introduced much faster during the long-term phases of the pandemic.[3] It needs to be acknowledged that many questions regarding the advantages and potential disadvantages of a wide telemedicine practice in sleep medicine remain to be fully understood.

CLINICAL APPLICATIONS AND FUTURE RESEARCH

Our data point toward several clinical implications. First, sleep medicine organizations are

Table 1
Studies analyzing the effects of COVID-19 pandemic on sleep medicine services

Type of Study	Country	Change in Diagnostic Procedures (% Change to Prepandemic Status)	Change in PAP Treatment of OSA (% Change to Prepandemic Status)	Comments
Questionnaire during early phase of pandemic[18]	19 European countries, 40 centers	−70%	−60%	Staffing levels reduced to 25% (physicians) and 19% (nurses). Insufficient use of telemedicine technologies
Questionnaire, posted 29th of April 2020 to AASM members[19]	297 sleep centers, 90% from the US	>90% reduction in activity: for PSG by 90.4% of centers, for HSAT by 60.3% of centers	>90% reduction in PSG-based PAP titration by 90.4% of centers	Reduced mask fitting procedures. Mitigation strategies: temperature testing, symptom evaluation, PCR testing; >70% virtual patient visits
Questionnaire during first 6 mo of 2020[20]	China, 56 sleep centers	Initially −90%, gradual improvement to −40%	Initially −95%, gradual improvement to −50%	
Description of sleep medicine service in New York during the COVID-19 outbreak spring 2020[21]	New York, descriptive data	PSG almost completely stopped, HSAT in selected cases	In-lab titration stopped, APAP used in selected patients	Use of HEPA filters and ventilated rooms in case of PAP titration procedures

Abbreviations: AASM, American Academy of Sleep Medicine; APAP, autotitrating positive airway pressure; HSAT, home sleep apnea testing; PSG, polysomnography, US, United States.

encouraged to monitor the status of sleep medicine services in their country as we were able to identify substantial regional differences. Second, strategies to maintain "practice as usual" need to be discussed on a regional and national level. Mitigation strategies to provide services should be considered not only in follow-up but also to undiagnosed or not-yet treated patients. Third, there is no current consensus on how to prioritize patients for sleep medicine services. Epidemiologic studies before the pandemic suggest that patients aged 65 years and younger may benefit from OSA treatment in terms of cardiovascular protection. On the other hand, mortality from COVID-19 is elevated in the elderly. Some experts recommend stopping PAP treatment due to aerosol contamination[5] and others propose high usage of all PAP

and bilevel PAP treatment of sleep-disordered breathing and the use of vented masks in case of infection.[3] Recommendations for both patients and caregivers based on strong scientific evidence should be available at all clinical sites. Indeed, there are now several guidance papers available on both national and international level published by the AASM,[1] the BTS,[2] the ERS,[3] the ITS,[23] the GAVO2,[4] or on national level.[5,6]

As fewer sleep studies are performed, fewer OSA cases are discovered, but the number of missed cases and the impact of the diagnostic delay cannot be assessed until after the pandemic. Another unresolved issue is how various health care systems will handle the increased inflow of new patients where treatment initialization is warranted once the pandemic is over. The ability of

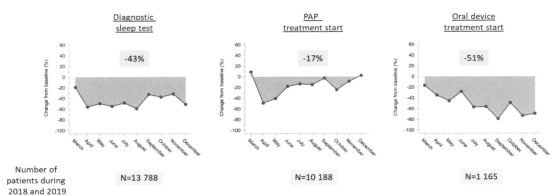

Fig. 4. Change in activities related to sleep apnea diagnosis and treatment during the first 10 months of the COVID-19 pandemic (March–December 2020). Numbers are based on the reported patient visits for each month (calculated as the change from the mean of 2018/2019). The blue area illustrates the reduction of activities during 2020. Only caregivers reporting during all 3 years are included in the analysis. The total number of patients for the different procedures is stated for 2018 and 2019. Data are presented as percentage change from baseline.

sleep centers to follow-up patients who are already receiving treatment may also be compromised in the long run. Despite several reports on increased PAP use during the pandemic,[24,25] low adherence is a known issue in PAP therapy, and a shift toward tele-medicine and a reduced access to physical visits treatment may systematically affect adherence. Although there are earlier intervention studies aiming at developing or testing the effects of telemedicine on PAP-adherence, they are typically performed in patients consenting to study participation. Findings from these studies cannot necessarily be generalized to a situation where a shift toward new routines is caused by a global pandemic. Some access to telemedicine interventions, such as video calls with a PAP therapy provider, also require fast Internet access, which may be less available to patients with lower socioeconomical background. It is therefore important to study whether socioeconomic factors may affect access to OSA diagnostics and treatment during and after the pandemic. Finally, the success of vaccination schemes in the general population may rapidly change the situation, and vaccination may be mandatory for at least some of the procedures performed in sleep centers. Many of those questions listed earlier cannot be fully examined until after the pandemic.

SUMMARY

The authors' findings suggest that the sleep medicine community needs to work together to develop strategies for care of patients with both suspected and established sleep-disordered breathing during major events such as the COVID-19 pandemic. Although personnel may be temporarily recruited to other areas of care,

remaining activities need to focus on the recognition of severe cases of SDB and initiate treatment in already identified severe cases. The potential of new technologies allowing for distant monitoring and optimization of treatment may be further used and developed during periods of limited health care resources outside the activities to manage severely affected patients with COVID-19.

CLINICS CARE POINTS

- Safety measures to avoid spread of the SARS-COV2 virus needs to be implemented when performing sleep diagnostic and therapeutic procedures in sleep centers to protect both personnel and patients. National and international guidance papers have been published.

- There is no firm evidence that untreated sleep apnea may increase the risk for severe COVID-19 with adverse outcome. However, successful treatment of severe sleep apnea is likely to be beneficial for patients with OSA when facing an acute SARS-COV2 infection.

- Patients with ongoing PAP therapy at home needs to be informed about the potential increased risk of virus spread for household members by PAP treatment in case of an acute infection. Use of humidifiers during PAP treatment need to be restricted to periods without symptoms of an SARS-COV2 infection.

- The use of telemedicine-based routines for diagnosis, treatment initiation, and follow up of patients with OSA has been implemented in many countries to overcome the partial lockdown of sleep medicine procedures. A large proportion of patients may have received equal or even improved sleep medicine services by telemedicine when compared with standard care before the pandemic. However, a subgroup of individuals needs more intensified personal contact with health care professionals. Personalized models of care need to be developed for sleep apnea management in the postpandemic period.

ACKNOWLEDGMENTS

The authors would like to acknowledge the support of the SESAR registry by Anna Nygren and Monika Hellstrand (register coordinators) and the statistical data analysis performed by Ludwig Andersson (statistician at Registercentrum Västra Götaland, Gothenburg). The authors also express our gratitude to the staff at the participating SESAR centers for continuous data entry during the study period, in particular during the circumstances of the COVID-19 pandemic.

DISCLOSURE

The authors have no conflict of interest to declare for the content of the submitted manuscript. Outside the submitted work, Dr L. Grote reports grants from Bayer, Philips Respironics Foundation, Resmed Foundation, European Respiratory Society, Itamar Medical, Resmed, and Philips. Dr L. Grote received personal fees for lectures from Respironics, Resmed, Itamar, Fisher &Paykel and Astra Zeneca. In addition. Dr L. Grote has two patents on sleep apnea therapy licensed.

REFERENCES

1. American Academy Sleep Medicine. COVID-19 mitigation strategies for sleep clinics and labs 2020. Available at: https://aasm.org/covid-19-resources/.

2. British Thoracic Society. Advice for those seeing patients with obstructive sleep apnoea. Available at: https://www.brit-thoracic.org.uk/about-us/covid-19-information-for-the-respiratory-community/.

3. Schiza S, Simonds A, Randerath W, et al. Sleep laboratories reopening and COVID-19: a European perspective. Eur Respir J 2021;57(3):2002722.

4. Gonzalez J, Maisonobe J, Oranger M, et al. GAVO2 procedures (French scientific group on chronic ventilation and oxygen) TITLE: homecare respiratory equipment for patients suspected to be infected with the respiratory virus Covid19 (English version). Version February 2020, French version updated April 2020. Available at: http://splf.fr/gavo2/.

5. Grote L, Albrecht D, Franklin K, et al. Vägledning angående coronavirus (COVID-19) och obstruktiv sömnapné (OSA). 2020. Available at: www.sesar.se/nyheter.

6. Grote L, Albrecht D, Friberg D, et al. Vägledning vid återstart av utredning och behandling av sömnapné under fortsatt COVID-19-pandemi- 2020. Available at: www.sesar.se/nyheter.

7. Baker JG, Sovani M. Case for continuing community NIV and CPAP during the COVID-19 epidemic. Thorax 2020;75(5):368.

8. Barker J, Oyefeso O, Koeckerling D, et al. COVID-19: community CPAP and NIV should be stopped unless medically necessary to support life. Thorax 2020;75(5):367.

9. Simonds A, Hanak A, Chatwin M, et al. Evaluation of droplet dispersion during non-invasive ventilation, oxygen therapy, nebuliser treatment and chest physiotherapy in clinical practice: implications for management of pandemic influenza and other airborne infections. Health Technol Assess 2010; 14(46):131–72.

10. B Benjafield AV, Ayas NT, Eastwood PR, et al. Estimation of the global prevalence and burden of obstructive sleep apnoea: a literature-based analysis. Lancet Respir Med 2019;7(8):687–98.

11. Bonsignore MR, Baiamonte P, Mazzuca E, et al. Obstructive sleep apnea and comorbidities: a dangerous liaison. Multidiscip Respir Med 2019;14:8.

12. Zhou F, Yu T, Du R, et al. Clinical course and risk factors for mortality of adult inpatients with COVID-19 in Wuhan, China: a retrospective cohort study. Lancet 2020;395(10229):1054–62.

13. Strausz S, Kiiskinen T, Broberg M, et al. Sleep apnoea is a risk factor for severe COVID-19. BMJ Open Respir Res 2021;8(1):e000845.

14. Oh TK, Song IA. Impact of coronavirus disease-2019 on chronic respiratory disease in South Korea: an NHIS COVID-19 database cohort study. BMC Pulm Med 2021;21(1):12.

15. Maas MB, Kim M, Malkani RG, et al. Obstructive sleep apnea and risk of COVID-19 infection, Hospitalization and respiratory failure. Sleep Breath 2020; 1–3. https://doi.org/10.1007/s11325-020-02203-0.

16. Goldstein CA, Rizvydeen M, Conroy DA, et al. The prevalence and impact of pre-existing sleep disorder diagnoses and objective sleep parameters in patients hospitalized for COVID-19. J Clin Sleep Med 2021. https://doi.org/10.5664/jcsm.9132.

17. Peker Y, Celik Y, Arbatli S, et al, OSACOVID-19 Study Collaborators. Effect of high-risk obstructive sleep apnea on clinical outcomes in adults with coronavirus disease 2019: a multicenter, prospective, observational cohort study. Ann Am Thorac Soc 2021. https://doi.org/10.1513/AnnalsATS.202011-1409OC.

18. Grote L, McNicholas WT, Hedner J, ESADA collaborators. Sleep apnoea management in Europe during the COVID-19 pandemic: data from the European sleep apnoea database (ESADA). Eur Respir J 2020;55(6):2001323.

19. Johnson KG, Sullivan SS, Nti A, et al. The impact of the COVID-19 pandemic on sleep medicine practices. J Clin Sleep Med 2021;17(1):79–87.

20. Zhang XL, Wang W, Xiao Y. Members of the assembly of sleep disordered breathing of the Chinese thoracic society. Sleep disordered breathing diagnosis and treatment during the COVID-19 pandemic: a nationwide survey in China. Nat Sci Sleep 2021;13:21–30.

21. Thorpy M, Figuera-Losada M, Ahmed I, et al. Management of sleep apnea in New York City during the COVID-19 pandemic. Sleep Med 2020;74: 86–90.

22. Sesar – Swedish sleep apnea registry- annual report 2019 (in Swedish). Available at: www.sesar.se. Accessed January 31, 2021.

23. Insalaco G, Dal Farra F, Braghiroli A, et al. A on behalf of the Italian thoracic society (ITS-AIPO): sleep breathing disorders in the COVID-19 era: Italian thoracic society organizational models for a correct approach to diagnosis and treatment. Respiration 2020;99(8):690–4.

24. Attias D, Pepin JL, Pathak A. Impact of COVID-19 lockdown on adherence to continuous positive airway pressure by obstructive sleep apnoea patients. Eur Respir J 2020;56(1):2001607.

25. Del Campo F, López G, Arroyo CA, et al. Study of the adherence to continuous positive airway pressure treatment in patients with obstructive sleep apnea Syndrome in the confinement during the COVID-19 pandemic. Arch Bronconeumol 2020;56(12):818–9.

Telemedicine in Sleep-Disordered Breathing
Expanding the Horizons

Johan Verbraecken, MD, PhD

KEYWORDS

- Telediagnosis • Telemonitoring • CPAP • Compliance • Telecounseling • Therapy reinforcement
- Behavior • Patient engagement

KEY POINTS

- Telemedicine has applications in all stages of the diagnosis, treatment, and follow-up of patients with sleep-disordered breathing. Diagnostic applications include telemonitored polysomnography, communication of test results and therapeutic options, and remote continuous positive airway pressure titration.
- Online compliance monitoring results in similar and in some cases improved compliance when compared with traditional face-to-face evaluations. The impact of telemedicine on compliance depends on the preexisting organization of standard care in the routine setting.
- Combining theory-driven behavioral approaches with telemedicine technology could hold the answer to increasing real-world adherence rates.
- Targeted troubleshooting and support based on individual patient data, web-, and/or app-based teaching, and combinations via a smartphone app or coaching website is feasible.
- Telemedicine is likely cost-effective but requires better evidence.

INTRODUCTION

Sleep medicine services have already undergone several disruptive changes related to new diagnostic and treatment technologies for the management of obstructive sleep apnea (OSA).[1,2] Telemedicine, the remote delivery of care with the use of technology, is an emerging field in the twenty-first century and has currently received widespread acceptance among diverse medical specialties across the globe thanks to the rapid proliferation of mobile and home-based devices.[3] Many sleep disorders are chronic conditions and require continuous treatment and monitoring of therapy success.[4] Telemedicine provides flexibility for using e-care in none, some, or many of the steps in OSA evaluation, diagnosis, and management.

Telemedicine-ready continuous positive airway pressure (CPAP) devices supporting the transmission of information on use time (hours per night), the apnea-hypopnea index (AHI), and leakage are available. The gathered data are sent via wireless networks to a secure server on the Internet, where it can be retrieved by the attending physician or sleep center. This opens new teleopportunities and e-opportunities for OSA care to replace, supplement, provide additional interim care and education, or improve practice workflows and costs for each of the different OSA treatments. Chronic management strategies, and big data deep learning applications may also be realized. With this, it is possible to serve patients better, to address problems early, and to inform on adverse side effects as well. In the end, this improves patient satisfaction and treatment adherence.

A recent position paper from the American Academy of Sleep Medicine related to the use of telemedicine in sleep disorders stressed that "the

Department of Pulmonary Medicine and Multidisciplinary Sleep Disorders Centre, Antwerp University Hospital, University of Antwerp, Drie Eikenstraat 655, Edegem, Antwerp 2650, Belgium
E-mail address: johan.verbraecken@uza.be

Sleep Med Clin 16 (2021) 417–445
https://doi.org/10.1016/j.jsmc.2021.05.009

practice of telemedicine should aim to promote a care model in which sleep specialists, patients, primary care providers, and other members of the healthcare team aim to improve the value of healthcare delivery in a coordinated fashion."[5]

Studies to date have used heterogeneous strategies and reported conflicting results.[6–10] Telehealth applications may be inserted in 1 or more of the workflow steps for diagnosis pathways, evaluation pathways, CPAP and non-CPAP treatments, and long-term follow-up. The current telemedicine applications are found to a smaller extent in the diagnostic procedures and to a much greater extent in the monitoring of therapy compliance for sleep apnea treatment. In this review, we will provide an overview of current practices, with the recent scientific progresses in telemonitoring for sleep-disordered breathing and their potential clinical applications for diagnosis and therapy, with emphasis on promising approaches to optimize adaptation and compliance:

- Diagnostic telemedicine applications: teletriage, telemonitored polysomnography (telesupervision, teletransmission), telecommunication of test results and treatment options
- Telemaskfitting and teleteaching (OSA and CPAP education)
- Tele CPAP titration
- Telemonitoring and problem solving:
  - Usual care
  - Remote monitoring CPAP therapy
  - Filter settings and fine-tuning of CPAP devices
- Telecounseling and therapy reinforcement: by combining and integrating the most promising elements of both psychoeducational interventions and technological innovations (active calls, digitized human speech, web-based access for patients to own CPAP data, automated messaging, and patient engagement tools)
- Telemanagement of comorbidities in OSA
- Telemedicine in particular populations
- Patient satisfaction and economic aspects (staff time, equipment, access to health care, addition of artificial intelligence, reimbursement, need for cost-benefit studies) will be highlighted.
- Changing paradigms and expanding horizons will be discussed.

Finally, also concerns related to telemedicine use and the remaining barriers and problems related to telemedicine implementation will also be addressed. In our opinion, all these telemedicine applications should be simple, with easy connectivity to external caregivers, achieving adequate training of nurses and physicians and should be directed to a specific group of patients.

DIAGNOSTIC TELEMEDICINE APPLICATIONS
Teletriage of Patients with Suspicion of Obstructive Sleep Apnea

Patients with OSA enter sleep center workflows through different pathways. Before testing and diagnosis, patients initially may be evaluated by the general physician, by somnologists or other specialists, or eventually by self-referral.[5,11,12] Proper identification for possible comorbid apnea conditions and inherent risks during the assessment and before testing is important in the choice of any OSA workflow path.[13] Telemedicine enables the documentation of baseline and follow-up OSA symptoms, sleepiness, quality of life, blood pressure, body mass index, comorbid disorders and traffic accident assessment, by making use of sleep medicine questionnaires that may be completed by patients through E-health patient portals, OSA risk assessment software or by phone.[14] Apart from the clinical guidelines for OSA test type, deep learning and artificial intelligence models using phenotyping, E-health record data, and other consumer or medical sensor devices and applications may provide insight for OSA risk assessment and test prioritization, or selection of tailored treatment paths.[15–19]

A thorough physical examination is not always possible when the patient is at home. In the assessment for possible OSA, tonsils can be difficult to estimate in size in 2-dimensional viewing. The clearest view of the oropharynx can be obtained if the patient or partner takes a photo on the smartphone and texts or emails it to the clinician. Also, the video from the camera on the back-side of the smartphone may be more likely to provide a clearer view of the oropharynx than the selfie view. Other important parts of the physical examination that are missing on virtual visits are overall appearance, evaluation of nasal turbinates, molar occlusion, heart, lungs, and eventually blood pressure. This difficulty can be overcome by creating special telemedicine hubs that include tools and equipment, including an intraoral camera, and a medical assistant who facilitates the transmission of this information.[20] Finally, coordination of care is more straightforward at the physical checkout counter, where appointments can be scheduled and paperwork can be printed and provided directly to the patient.

Telediagnosis (Teletransmission, Telesupervision)

Telemonitored polysomnography (PSG) has the premise to overcome the disadvantages of home recordings and could provide an organizational solution to the overloading of specialized sleep centers. Telemedicine can be used in the context of sleep studies for 2 purposes.[21] The first is to facilitate swift transmission of data of home PSG for further analysis. The second purpose for the application of telemedicine for sleep recording has been to ensure the quality of unattended PSG, by intermittent or continuous remote supervision of recording. Dedicated technicians regularly verify, at a distance, the quality of the PSG recordings by means of periodic access to the PSG monitoring device. From their telemonitoring control panel, they are able to insert comments in the recording, adjust transducer gain and, in the event of an artifact or an undesirable accident (disconnected wires, misplaced equipment), inform the patient by telephone.[22] However, evidence on the efficacy of telemonitored (P)SG is weak. Gagnadoux and colleagues[23] reported that PSG performed in a local hospital and telemonitored by a sleep laboratory was clearly superior to unattended home PSG. Kristo and colleagues[24] proposed a telemedicine protocol for the online transfer of PSGs from a remote site to a centralized sleep laboratory, that had practitioners for diagnosis, which provided a cost-saving approach for the diagnosis of OSA. Their system was based on the transmission of data using an Internet FTP protocol, which is the conventional system for file transfer. Kayyali and colleagues[25] presented a new compact telemetry-based sleep monitor (PSG@Home), consisting of a 14-channel wearable wireless monitor and a cell phone-based Gateway to transfer data, including video, in real time from the patient's home to a remote sleep center. The monitor can easily be worn and transported, and it offers reliable recordings.[25] The receiver is a separate unit connected with the back of the display. Internal Bluetooth receivers, usually included in laptops, can also be used instead of a dedicated external Bluetooth receiver. A major problem encountered with home sleep studies is the potential loss of data in about 4.7% to 20.0% of the cases, which results in lower than expected cost savings.[26] Using Sleepbox technology (Medatec, Brussels, Belgium), a wireless system able to communicate with the polysomnograph and with Internet through a WiFi/3G interface, and communicating via Skype, the authors were able to deliver recordings with excellent quality in 90% of the cases.[27] This opens an interesting perspective to decrease the failure rate of home sleep studies, although still problematic, and some technical aspects need to be improved. Pelletier-Fleury and colleagues[28] comparatively evaluated the cost and effectiveness of PSG telemonitoring and PSG by conventional unsupervised home monitoring, and demonstrated that remote telemonitoring made the procedure clearly superior from a technical point of view and was preferred by the patients. They obtained a cost of \$US244 for PSG telemonitoring, whereas the PSG with conventional unsupervised home monitoring was \$US153. The health care infrastructure savings have to be taken into account as well. If we add up the working days that the patients did not lose and the roundtrip travel costs they avoided, we could estimate that the real cost would be similar or lower than that of conventional PSG.[29] Placement of polygraphy was performed by the local nursing staff, under remote supervision from a central sleep laboratory, in patients likely to suffer from OSA. Continuous video monitoring via a webcam was also included.[29] Masa and colleagues[30] compared the costs made between device transportation and telematic transmission of data, with comparable results. Having devices moved by a transportation company or sent telematically as raw data proved cost effective and equally beneficial. Borsini and colleagues[31] from Buenos Aires performed polygraphy at home, but fitted by nonexpert technicians. Raw data were sent by e-mail to the sleep center the following day. The failure rate was 4%, and 12% needed an additional in-laboratory PSG.

These positive results can allow health care providers to enhance accessibility to sleep tests in large countries with few expert sleep centers and for patients who live a long way from the hospital or those with limited mobility.[30,31] Fields and colleagues[32] demonstrated the feasibility of a comprehensive, telemedicine-based OSA evaluation and management pathway in comparison with a more traditional, in-person care model. They combined video consultation for intake with home sleep testing using a type 3 portable monitor with remote download, and autoCPAP titration with wireless modem technology. Patient satisfaction, CPAP adherence, and compliance and improvement in quality of life was similar in both groups.

Although not applied routinely in current practice, these studies have confirmed the feasibility and the potential interest in telemonitored sleep studies. Moreover, this approach to diagnosis is considered to be more convenient for the patient than staying at a clinic overnight. The widespread use of telediagnosis is slowed down by the costs and the complexity of the technical aspects, and also requires a change to the current model of care delivery, because as it will become patient and home centered, rather than hospital centered. Such disruptive changes are going to take time to be effectuated.

New Simplified Diagnostic Telemedicine Applications

In clinical practice, the use of PSG is a standard procedure to assess sleep-disordered breathing. However, PSG is not suitable for chronic monitoring in the home environment and not very convenient to the patient. New telemedicine applications have become available using a home appliance as a precautionary measure for monitoring snoring and OSA. Seo and colleagues[33] developed a nonintrusive health monitoring home system to monitor patients' ECG results, weight, motor activity, and snoring. Choi and colleagues[34] proposed a ubiquitous health monitoring system in a bedroom, which monitors the electrocardiogram, body movements, and snoring with nonconscious sensors. Böhning and colleagues[35] evaluated the feasibility of night-time pulse oximetry telemedicine to screen patients at risk for OSA. They concluded the technique seemed to be suitable and cost effective, with high sensitivity and specificity. This approach can be applied in a telemedicine referral network for early diagnosis of OSA, where the reading could be transmitted to the relevant sleep laboratory, examined, and the results returned to the referring physician.[36]

Of note, several consumer device technologies with pulse oximetry, heart rate variability, actigraphy and deep learning algorithms are undergoing US Food and Drug Administration evaluation as home sleep apnea testing devices.[37]

Devices available today offer a wireless transmission of recording modules to the main body unit worn at the chest (by Blue-tooth technology), also called body area network.[38] In some cases, a Bluetooth application can be used to send data to a smartphone or a tablet for online continuous monitoring. Also, the storage of data is wireless by making use of cloud-based storing.[4]

Telecommunication of Test Results and Treatment Options

In line with OSA best practice and quality measure guidelines, the communication of the test results and treatment options with the patient may be done at face-to-face visits or using telemedicine tools such as videoconferencing, teleconferencing, and e-health portal messaging.[32] In Spain, Coma-del-Corral and colleagues[29] applied teleconsultation in patients with confirmed OSA. After a telemonitored polygraphy, patients were randomised to receive either a teleconsultation or a face-to-face consultation to receive the results of their sleep study. The teleconsultation was organized via video conferencing. In those patients that finally were treated with CPAP, adherence was not different between the groups: 85% for the face-to-face consultation and 75% for the teleconsultation group. In many telehealth services, there is considerable variation in who communicates the test results to patients, among them somnologists or other specialists, nurses, physician assistants, sleep laboratory technicians, respiratory therapists, noninvasive ventilation therapists, or other trained staff.[5,19,32,39] The impact of communicating test results cannot enough be emphasized. When patients view results of their diagnostic study with an explanation of the frequency and duration of respiratory events, it results in increased compliance of 0.7 to 1.2 hours per night on average.[40–42] Clinicians can show raw data and trends from the PSG virtually by the share screen feature to visually explain the extent and severity of the sleep-disordered breathing.

TELETHERAPY
Tele-Mask Fitting and Teleteaching (Obstructive Sleep Apnea and Continuous Positive Airway Pressure)

In standard care, CPAP setup and teaching is offered by trained sleep technicians and respiratory therapists, which is recognized to be labor intensive, but critical for final compliance. Switching to video CPAP setups and remote education may offer decreased labor time while maintaining improved or equivalent CPAP compliance and satisfaction.[5] Facial recognition software, application of mask sizers, mask fit packs and artificial intelligence analysis of mask fitting selection phenotypes may support remote CPAP mask selection and setup options.[43] Although early educational interventions before CPAP initiation are strongly recommended, the effect of tele-education alone on overall compliance does not seem robust, which could be explained by confounding factors such as the variability of the initial and following tele-education deliveries, and easy availability of Internet-based OSA and CPAP educational resources for patients with OSA.[44] Different authors found improved compliance for patients given Web access to their data and companion educational resources.[45–47] Smith and colleagues[48] tested a teleconferencing approach in which a nurse visually assessed mask fit and patients' CPAP procedures and provided counseling and reinforcement to patients who were trying CPAP again after an initial 3-month period of poor compliance. Although the patient education materials supplied during the initial period did not impact adherence rates, the nurse teleconferencing sessions during the second trial period substantially improved the adherence of the intervention group (9 of 10 patients vs 4 of 9 in the placebo intervention group), suggesting that intensity of one-on-one counseling and feedback by a care provider is a relevant variable.[48] Isetta and colleagues[49] performed a randomized controlled trial (RCT) in which 20 patients with OSA received standard face-to-face training, and another 20 received the CPAP training via videoconference. Patients demonstrated comparable knowledge about OSA and CPAP therapy, while performance of practical skills (mask and headgear placement, leak avoidance) and knowledge related to OSA was also similar between the 2 groups (94% correct answers in the videoconference groups vs 92%).[49] In another study of the same group in 139 patients with OSA, similar levels of CPAP compliance, and improved daytime sleepiness, quality of life, side effects and degree of satisfaction was found in a telemedicine-based CPAP follow-up strategy (televisits via video conference based on Skype, e-mail, web tool support) compared with face-to-face management.[50] Interestingly, the telemedicine group made more extra visits than the face-to-face group, but most of them were not OSA related.

Tele Continuous Positive Airway Pressure Titration

An exploratory study was set up to perform real-time titration of domiciliary CPAP.[51] The novelty of this approach is that a telemetry unit is connected to a commercially available CPAP device to allow a low-cost, 2-way communication channel in real time between the sleep laboratory technician and the CPAP device in the patient's home. The approach requires no special telemedicine approach, nor does it require the patient's active cooperation or any kind of communication infrastructure (computer or the Internet) in the patient's home. This interesting exploratory study allowed sleep technicians to avoid potential failures of automatic positive airway pressure (APAP) trials at home. Unfortunately, no larger scale trials have been performed. However, in times of home-APAP titration, it can be wondered whether it is really necessary to obtain a remote real-time control of titration. In contrast, a routine visit to the hospital shortly after home APAP titration to check the CPAP device data can be avoided with a remote-attended titration strategy. A barrier to this approach could be related to the contraindications rather than to technical aspects. In our local experience, the proportion of patients who can benefit from home APAP titration is less than 40% (unpublished data). The presence of comorbidities (neuropsychiatric, cardiorespiratory comorbidities and comorbid insomnia and morbid obesity) also restricts access to this pathway.[52] Nevertheless, it permits flexibility in resetting the therapy remotely through online pressure adjustments as clinically needed.[52–54]

Telemonitoring of Continuous Positive Airway Pressure Compliance and Adherence and Problem Solving

Usual care (or standard care)

Because CPAP is a self-administered treatment, its efficacy is critically dependent on the patient's willingness to use the device and apply the nasal mask during sleep, regardless of how well a CPAP machine corrects apnea. In this context, the term adherence is used to describe continued use of the machine (uptake), and compliance expresses the use of CPAP for a certain amount of time.[55] Unfortunately, these terms are often inadequately used and mutually exchanged. A user is defined as a patient that uses his device for more than 4 hours per night. Commonly used definitions of adequate compliance are use of more than 4 hours per night for 70% of days or more than 4 hours per night for more than 5 days per week.[56,57]

Early compliance (at 1 week or 1 month) is associated with better compliance at 6 months, indicating that early interventions and support should be offered to patients.[58]

Different studies have shown that the rates of CPAP use are between 30% and 60%. Of importance, patients who become nonadherent in the first days of CPAP treatment generally remain nonadherent.[59] Without optimal CPAP use, patients will fail to achieve the full cardiovascular and symptomatic benefits of therapy. Hence, compliance for CPAP should be regarded as the main determinant for success.[55] Usually, the patient is seen by a qualified sleep professional to assess CPAP use (hours of use and hours of application), to check the machine settings, and to ensure the interface (mask, pillows, and so forth) is in good condition. Short-term and long-term follow-up are crucial to adherence and compliance, but monitoring efficacy is also critical to adherence, compliance, and successful therapy. In one study, compliance monitoring, including consistent follow-up, troubleshooting, and feedback to both patients and physicians, achieved good CPAP compliance rates (>4 hours per night) of more than 80% over 6 months.[60] In contrast, close follow-up has not been consistently shown to improve compliance, but is worth doing.[49] Even more effective is to establish adherence and compliance patterns early in treatment initiation, which can help to resolve problems in a timely manner and is essential in the effort to establish a pattern of treatment adherence and good compliance.[61] Intervention early in therapy may improve the patient's early response to CPAP therapy and increase the likelihood that the patient will become a regular and compliant user, thereby enhancing clinical outcome. CPAP follow-up appointments vary from 3 months to yearly, according to physician preferences and availability of resources, without check-ups between follow-up visits. For those patients who are doing well with their current therapy, the annual compliance visit may deliver little value because many visits are not associated with any meaningful changes in management.[62] This model results in lost time at work for patients, decreased productivity for their employers, and less space in a busy clinician's agenda to manage more complex patients.[29,50,63] Finally, it can be frustrating for patients and clinicians when the patient is seen in office yet forgets to bring their problematic mask, tubing, or machine.

Rationale for improving compliance

The challenge with CPAP therapy is to obtain adequate adherence and compliance, usually defined as use of CPAP during at least 4 hours per night and for more than 70% of the nights.[64] This threshold is somewhat arbitrary and has been debated because a dose–response relationship between PAP use and clinical outcomes in OSA has been demonstrated. However, there is general acknowledgment that more is better with respect to CPAP use. A systematic review of 66 clinical trials and cohort studies published between 1994 and 2015 found a weighted average compliance of 4.5 hours per night, with no meaningful improvement in compliance rates over the 2 decades of data available since objective CPAP monitoring was introduced.[65] The literature to date suggests a dose–response relationship between CPAP use and a range of outcomes, including sleepiness, functional status, and blood pressure. Weaver and colleagues[64] could demonstrated that when using the Functional Outcomes of Sleep Questionnaire, a greater improvement in memory was obtained when CPAP was used more than 6 hours per night in comparison with less than 2 hours. In a Spanish study, Barbé and

colleagues[66] demonstrated in a cohort of 359 patients with OSA that nightly use longer than 5.65 hours achieved better blood pressure and sleepiness reduction. Gasa and colleagues[67] reported that the prevalence of residual excessive sleepiness is significantly lower in individuals using CPAP more than 6 hours per night compared with those who use the device less than 4 hours per night (8.7% vs 18.5%). A recent randomized study in a cohort of 3100 CPAP-treated patients, randomized in intensive versus standard interventions, also confirmed the positive effect of a greater CPAP use (6.9 vs 5.2 hours per night) on cardiovascular outcomes, indicating that a regular 5 to 6 hours of use per night is required.[68] In a recent Cochrane Database Systematic Review that pooled data from 30 low-to-moderate quality studies it was reported that supportive, educational, and behavioral therapy increases compliance by a respective amount of 50, 35, and 104 minutes per night, resulting in a greater proportion of patients using CPAP for more than 4 hours per night.[69] A meta-analysis of 12 trials (572 patients) concluded that each 1-hour improvement in CPAP compliance was associated with a reduction in mean blood pressureof 1.4 mm Hg.[70] Bratton and colleagues[71] showed that a 1-hour per night increase in mean CPAP use was associated with an additional decrease in the systolic blood pressure of 1.5 mm Hg and an additional reduction in diastolic blood pressure of 0.9 mm Hg. CPAP compliance is usually defined as simply hours per night rather than as a proportion of total sleep time, which is usually not measured.[72] Therefore, it is unclear as to whether short sleep duration (eg, 4 h) with 100% CPAP compliance would lead to greater impairment than longer sleep duration (eg, 8 h) with 50% CPAP compliance, even though the CPAP use is identical in both instances. Finally, suboptimal CPAP use has prevented a thorough understanding of important trials designed to clarify the impact of OSA on cardiovascular risk and the role of CPAP in mitigating that risk.[73,74]

(Cloud-based) remote compliance monitoring: Technical aspects

Many CPAP devices have an integrated digital storage to record patient use data, which allows to download previously recorded data.[10,48,60,75] It allows recording with little subject interference under normal and experimental conditions.[4] CPAP devices are now equipped with simple global system for mobile communication modules to transmit exactly these use and aggregated diagnostic data to medical service providers. Patients can transmit CPAP data on a daily basis into a database (eg, the Encore Anywhere database, Philips; ResTraxx database, ResMed), where data extraction takes place. Because PAP manufacturers use proprietary cloud-based data platforms and use different algorithms for respiratory event detection, this can be a potential non–patient-related barrier to telemedicine adoption (**Table 1**). As a result, health care professionals may require access to several different databases and because not all patients use the same brand of CPAP devices, technical standards are needed to enable aggregation into one's health care record.[47] In the past, a universal telemonitoring unit was available (T4P, SRETT Medical, France), which offered the possibility to be added to the majority of CPAP devices, and to be switched from one patient to another for a determined duration, according to the patient needs.[76] This system also made use of a telemedicine web platform (T4P Vision Web Portal) that was the same for all patients. Unfortunately, the company does not exist anymore. Another universal telemonitoring unit is called NOWAPI, but is poorly examined.[77] An apnea was considered when a tidal volume of less than 20% of the patient reference tidal volume was detected (for $\geq$10s), whereas a hypopnea was counted if a tidal volume between 20% and 50% of the patient reference tidal volume was found (for $\geq$10 s). Of interest, there was a concern related to low satisfaction rate of the patients about the traffic light indicator.

Fine tuning of continuous positive airway pressure devices and filter settings for interventions during telemonitoring

One of the capabilities of telemedicine is probably the early detection of problems (such as persistent respiratory events or leakage), thus facilitating appropriate interventions, and thereby improving the patients early experience with CPAP.[39] Hoet and colleagues[76] showed that telemonitoring significantly reduced the delay to the first intervention for CPAP treatment (29 $\pm$ 25 vs 47 $\pm$ 30 days). For this purpose, the data have to be analyzed against a set of preestablished criteria or filters. The dataset can be scanned for multiple criteria and compared with thresholds for adherence and compliance, trends, AHI, periodic breathing, occurrence of central apneas and mask leaks.[77]

A selection of filter settings reported in the literature or by companies is shown in **Table 2**.[6,7,76,78,79,80,81]

For example, CPAP data are automatically sent to the health care provider on a daily basis and trigger automatic alarms in case of poor use for 2 consecutive nights (<4 h) or excessive mask leakage (>0.5 L/s).[81] Automatically triggered clinical actions can then be scheduled (**Fig. 1**). The final goal of such a platform is to proactively identify and address issues that can negatively influence CPAP adherence and compliance. By providing patient data early in the course of CPAP treatment, it is believed that this technology would be extremely useful in improving compliance and acceptance of the device in patients with sleep apnea.[9,10,48,75,82–86] All that is needed is a personal computer, an Internet connection, and the proprietary software. Detailed reports can be generated to show use information and then forwarded electronically to referral laboratories or physicians without generating additional paperwork. Wireless applications with an in-built telemonitoring module connects the CPAP unit in the patient's home with a server each evening

Table 1
Problems with the platforms for CPAP telemonitoring

Problem	Comment
Communication protocol depends on manufacturer	Ideally, communication software should adapt to different manufacturers. In practice, a universal system is not feasible, also taking into account the implementation of data encryption by the communication device.
Type and quality of measured data depend on manufacturer's technology	PAP devices detect snoring and respiratory events by airway pressure vibrations or flow changes.
Detection of respiratory events is dictated by algorithms developed by the PAP manufacturer	Criteria for respiratory events are based on the magnitude reduction of the flow signal (<50% for hypopneas; <10% for apneas). However, baseline value is not adequately defined and even does not remain constant during sleep.

Table 2
Proposed filter settings for interventions during telemonitoring

	Compliance	Leaks	Residual AHI
Fox et al,[6] 2012	<4 h use on 2 consecutive days (check every week day)	Mask leak >40 L/min for >30% of the night	>10 events/h, and 90th percentile of pressure >16 cm H_2O
Frasnelli et al,[78] 2016	<4 h use on 2 consecutive days	>30 L/min for more than 2 d	Not included
Munafo et al,[7] 2016	No CPAP data for 2 consecutive days <4 h use for 3 consecutive days	>30 L/min for >2 d	>15/h for 5 consecutive days
Chumpangern et al,[79] 2021	<4 h use on 2 consecutive days	>27 L/min on 2 consecutive days	>5/h on 2 consecutive days
Hoet et al,[76] 2017	<3 h use on 3 consecutive days	>50 L/min	>10/h
Turino et al,[80] 2017	<4 h use on 2 consecutive days	>30 L/min for >30% of the night	NA
Prigent et al,[81] 2020	<4 h use over a period of 7 consecutive days. During the initiation period: compliance check each 72 h	1 h of relevant leaks (Philips) Nonintentional leaks: ith 95th percentile >24 L/min (nasal mask ResMed) With 95th percentile >36 L/min (oronasal mask ResMed) Overall leakage >60 L/min (Fisher and Paykel) Overall leakage of >95 L/min (Devilbiss) Nonintentional leaks with a mean ≥ 20 L/min Nonintentional leaks with 95th percentile ≥60 L/min Percent elevated leakage ≥15% (Löwenstein) ≥5% of the use time above the leakage limit (Sefam)	≥10/h in a progressive window of 7 d

and transmits adherence and compliance data on a daily base. This technology eliminates the need for data cards or home telephone lines, and frequent patient visits. The compliance server analyzes the data and notifies the physician of any patients with poor CPAP use. Patient confidentiality is secured through a password and login-protected system that provides protection for the patients' information. Such system provides accurate, thorough, and advanced information to the clinician and ensures that each patient is receiving the maximum benefit from CPAP therapy. A patient's own data can be checked at a glance with physician summary reports. Visual color coding allows the caregiver to easily identify patients who require attention. Remote settings changes are available to fine tune therapy and optimize patient management. Historical data can be searched at any time to retrieve data that were not transmitted via the monitoring schedule. Telemonitoring of CPAP data may enable early identification of central sleep apnea or Cheyne–Stokes breathing and congestive heart failure occurrence or progression.[39,87] This technology has the potential also to be used for noninvasive ventilation in other types of patients and in more advanced devices for respiratory support.[88] Telemonitoring may be useful in patients with sleep apnea who

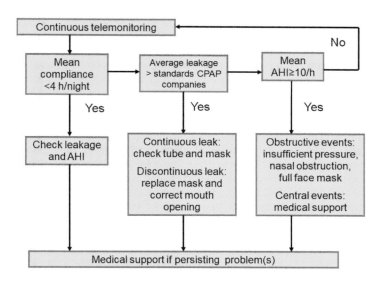

Fig. 1. A decision tree for telemonitoring of PAP therapy.

require other modes of PAP therapy. Patients with noninvasive ventilation require a much closer therapy control protocol compared with patients with sleep apnea.

One of the drawbacks of CPAP unit residual AHI is that this parameters is based on recording time and may include snoring and vibration in the total residual event calculation (CPAP AHI is not similar to PSG AHI).[89,90]

Again, we have to take into account that major differences exist between manufacturer definitions of residual events (see **Table 1**) and that an AHI flow is not associated with nonadherence.[90–92] The key advantage of this technology is that the individual's CPAP data are now automatically collected, remotely accessible, and actionable by both providers and patients.[93] However, it suffers from the limitation that it leads to data overload when trying to manage a large patient population.

Fine tuning of continuous positive airway pressure devices: Responsibilities

If such a feature is implemented, additional regulations have to be considered. Who is liable if the pressure adjustment is not functioning properly? Is this a matter of data transmission, or was the device in use with another patient? Before bidirectional telemedicine is implemented in the therapy of sleep apnea on a large scale, several legal questions need to be clarified.[4] Roles, expectations, and responsibilities of providers involved in the delivery of such services should be defined and communicated, including those at originating sites and distant sites.[5] The assumptions parties may have in such encounters and roles should be explicitly documented. In general, the standards

for supervision should follow the same general guidelines as those for technicians, respiratory care practitioners, and nurses working with physicians in the live setting. All providers involved have to review their facilities' and institutions' bylaws and human resource documents. Moreover, relevant regulatory documents related to the provision of care are to be followed, and organizations and providers are to ensure such care is consistent with policies regarding scope of practice and state licensing laws of all involved parties.[5,94] However, it is questionable whether a service provider could be allowed to fine tune CPAP settings independently, because changing treatment regimens is the physician's privilege and responsibility for centuries. To overcome this problem, the physician must be available by telephone to provide assistance and direction if needed. Telemedicine could be readily used to augment general supervision, and asynchronous methods could be used.[5] One more barrier, in some countries, is that CPAP fitting and troubleshooting is not eligible for reimbursement, when performed via telemedicine by respiratory therapists and sleep technologists.[95] Who gets access to these data with personal use information also varies from country to country according to local medical data regulations. Some countries regulations are very restrictive and require a clear distinction of tasks among health Insurance, service provider, and sleep physician.

(Cloud-based) remote compliance monitoring: evidence

Unlike pill-based treatments, CPAP is unique in that detailed, night-by-night compliance data are collected routinely and can be made available in real time to both patients and providers.

Some study results suggest that the use of tele-monitored CPAP compliance and efficacy data seems to be as good as standard care in its effect on compliance rates and outcomes in new CPAP users, although conflicting data remain.[10,96,97] However, the results from other RCTs regarding improvement in compliance are disappointing (**Table 3**), given many studies do not show any improvement in compliance with telemonitoring. In contrast, in some of these studies, despite the application of telemonitoring, compliance remained extremely low, questioning the level of usual care in these centers.[6,9] Nevertheless, tele-monitoring offers the possibility for the sleep medicine providers to detect "problematic" patient and to act properly. Stepnowsky and colleagues[10] demonstrated that a telemonitored clinical care group had a compliance rate of 4.1 hours per night after 2 months, which represents a 46% increase in compliance over the mean compliance level of the standard clinical care group (2.8 hours per night). However, this trial was certainly underpowered to reach significance ($P<.07$) but provided a rationale for conducting larger clinical and cost-effectiveness trials. There were also some concerns regarding the potential loss of data through wireless transmission. However, the loss was negligible and once the wireless unit was properly connected, data from previous nights stored on the flow generator device could be retransmitted and obtained wirelessly. Anttalainen and colleagues[98] compared a group of wireless telemonitored CPAP users with a usual care group, after CPAP titration. They found equal CPAP compliance and residual AHI at the 1-year follow up. The median nursing time was 39 minutes in the telemonitored group and shorter compared with that of 58 minutes per patient in the usual care group. Fernandes and colleagues[103] reported that in the presence of a comprehensive educational program during positive airway pressure adaptation, telemonitoring patients did not show significant benefits concerning compliance and efficacy. A larger follow-up period was proposed to evaluate the long-term results of a telemonitoring program.

Long-term follow-up

Because OSA may change with aging, weight, menopause, and intake of some medications, long-term OSA monitoring for all treatments is indicated.[106,107] Studies confirmed the feasibility of tel-econsultation as a parallel route to face-to-face consultations, not only during the critical CPAP habituation phase, but also on the long run. This type of telemedicine seems to be easier to practice, because it does not require changes in the model of care delivery, just a pragmatic teleconference platform. This approach is associated with numerous advantages for patients, including the removal of the need to travel to and from the sleep medicine center. Baig and colleagues[108] demonstrated the long-term effectiveness of a 5-year telemedicine program: the delay to obtain CPAP was reduced from more than 2 months to less than 1 week, the total number of sleep consultations decreased, and the waiting list time for the sleep clinic shortened. Murphie and colleagues. reported high satisfaction in a Scottish cohort, and Isetta and colleagues found similar satisfaction rates after video-based PAP follow-up encounters.[49,109]

In contrast, the limitation of synchronous telemedicine is that it still requires face-to-face provider time, and its impact on care efficiency is modest at the best.[93] To be so, it requires adoption of elements that largely fall under the umbrella of asynchronous telemedicine. Parikh and colleagues[63] compared teleconsultation delivered by video conferencing with face-to-face consultation for follow-up of CPAP therapy in 90 patients. The proportion of compliant patients and levels of patient satisfaction were not different between the 2 groups. Nevertheless, the ideal frequency of face-to-face follow-up for maintenance of CPAP adherence remains to be elucidated. Murase and colleagues[105] could demonstrate a favorable effect of a telemedicine intervention on treatment adherence in long-term CPAP users, and found that visits every 3 months with a monthly telemedicine intervention had a beneficial change in adherence similar to monthly visits. This finding may suggest that telemedicine interventions can assume some of the merits of close face-to-face follow-up for the maintenance of CPAP adherence. No improvement was found in CPAP compliance data. Because those participants were familiar with using CPAP, they probably appreciated the decrease in the number of clinic visits. The greater level of satisfaction in the telemedicine group may be a strong rationale to promote this approach.

Telemedicine monitoring of sleep apnea therapy is currently limited to CPAP and related ventilator-support devices. However, alternative treatment modalities are coming in place, like mandibular advancement device and sleep position trainers. For example, it has been shown that mandibular advancement devices can be monitored objectively as well by in-built thermosensors, with wireless transmission of adherence and compliance data.[110] For these devices, ongoing remote data monitoring of adherence is needed as well. However, the frequency of follow-up testing for these

Table 3
Randomized studies comparing telemedicine monitoring versus standard care in CPAP therapy

	N	AHI	Telemonitoring Method	Follow-up	Compliance TM	Compliance UC	P Value
Taylor et al,[75] 2006	114	>5	Internet support + feedback	1 mo	4.3 h	4.2 h	NS
Stepnowsky et al,[10] 2007	45	>15	Interactive web site with own CPAP data and instructions for troubleshooting	2 mo	4.1 h	3.4 h	S
Sparrow et al,[9] 2010	250	>10	Interactive voice response system	6 mo	2.4 h	1.48 h	S
Fox et al,[6] 2012	75	>15	Feedback by phone	3 mo	3.2 h	1.7 h	S
Isetta et al,[50] 2015	139	Mean 49	Feedback by webtools	6 mo	4.4 h	4.2 h	NS
Anttalainen et al,[98] 2016	111	Mean 34	Nurse-adjusted phone/visits	12 mo	6.4 h	6.1 h	NS
Frasnelli et al,[78] 2016	223	37 (TM) 40 (UC)	Telemonitoring and messaging	1 mo	53 h	4.6 h	S
Munafo et al,[7] 2016	132	34 (TM) 27 (UC)	Multimedia approach to contact patient about their CPAP use	1 mo	5.1 h	4.7 h	NS
Turino et al,[80] 2017	140	52 (TM) 53 (UC)	Telemonitoring	3 mo	5.1 h	4.9 h	NS
Hostler et al,[99] 2017	61	19 (TM) 18 (UC)	Telemonitoring, patient engagement tool	11 wk	4.0 h	2.7 h	NS
Hwang et al,[44] 2018	1455	23 (TM) 23 (TE) 22 (UC)	Telemonitoring, messaging, web-based OSA education	3 mo	4.8 h	3.8	S
Hoet et al,[76] 2017	46	50 (TM) 49 (UC)	Telemonitoring	3 mo	5.7	4.2	S
Kotzian et al,[100] 2019	33	37 (TM) 37 (UC)	CPAP training + monitoring	3 mo 12 mo	6.3 h 5.9 h	5.0 h 5.1 h	S NS
Nilius et al,[101] 2019	80	41 (TM) 38 (UC)	Short telephone calls	6 mo	4.4 h	2.1 h	S
Pépin et al,[102] 2019	306	47 (TM) 45 (UC)	Multimodal telemonitoring Home blood pressure and physical activity	6 mo	5.28 h	4.75 h	S
Fernandes et al,[103] 2019	51	38 (TM) 36 (UC) 36 (PC)	Remote monitoring and intervention	4 wk	5.0 h	5.1 h	NS
Schoch et al,[8] 2019	240	37 (TM) 46 (UC)	Remote monitoring and phone calls	6 mo	5.6 h	4.8 h	NS
Tamisier et al,[104] 2020	206	45 (TM) 42 (UC)	Multimodal telemonitoring	6 mo	4.73 h	5.08 h	NS
Murase et al,[105] 2020	483	161 (TM) 166 (UC)	Remote monitoring and phone calls	6 mo	5.45	5.12	NS
Chumpangern et al,[79] 2021	57	49 (TM) 52 (UC)	Remote monitoring and intervention	4 wk	5.16	4.42	NS

Abbreviations: NS, not significant; S, significant; TM, telemonitoring; UC, usual care.

non-CPAP therapies does not seem clear. Altogether, telemedicine technologies could change the classical visits toward an outside clinic visit program, with shorter and more frequent visits realized by different communication methods.

PATIENT COUNSELING AND THERAPY REINFORCEMENT

The use of telemedicine has the ability to quickly collect, transmit, and incorporate data, making it a swift and viable means of communication between patients and their providers.[111] These features have a significant potential for the management of patients with OSA, particularly for education and counseling, apart from optimizing CPAP adherence and close monitoring of effective compliance. This type of intervention also has the added potential benefit of fostering patient empowerment. Patients who take ownership, who are involved in their own care, and possess the knowledge and skills to manage their disease are more likely to comply with lifestyle modifications and treatment regimens, which in turn improves clinical outcomes.[112] In this way, telemedicine can have a substantial impact on health care use, strengthen the sleep professional–patient interaction, and enhance self-management skills.[113]

Patient Counseling and Personalized Feedback (Video and Teleconferencing)

Video and telephone contacts provide both direct and indirect benefits to patients. Direct benefits include decreased waiting time, and increased physician availability. Indirect benefits include avoidance of barriers to in-person visits, such as the cost and time associated with travel or missed work.[114] Video visits could accommodate chronic routine follow-up appointments. Patient specific data, such as diaries for insomnia and CPAP machine downloads for OSA, could be reviewed at such visits, as could routine challenges with equipment or medications.[114] As mentioned elsewhere in this article, a concern could be that the doctor might need to perform some physical examination. However, in sleep medicine it may be that stable patients could be adequately assessed without performing a physical examination that requires the physician to be present in the same room. In addition, certain elements of the examination, such as weight or blood pressure measurement could be performed at home or by the family physician. In a series of 90 patients with OSA, 56 were seen by a physician at the sleep center and 34 by videoconference. Satisfaction did not differ between the groups.[63] A successful telemedicine encounter should mirror the live visits as much

as possible.[95] Therefore, close attention should be paid to the technical quality of the encounter, starting with the video and audio specifications.

Video teleconferencing may improve access to care without compromising important clinical outcomes. Cost and provider time analyses have not been not undertaken so far.

Promotion and Reinforcement of Patient Adherence and Compliance

The optimal use of CPAP requires a level of patient engagement that exceeds what is needed to follow a pill-based regimen. Although teaching is likely necessary to provide foundational knowledge for behavior change, information may not be enough to induce significant and sustained behavior changes. Also, it can be questioned whether technology-based delivery of education can be a more cost-effective approach. Instead, addition of motivational elements such as personalized goal setting or other methods such as accountability may be essential.

Behavioral determinants explain up to approximately 20% of the total variance in CPAP compliance emphasizing the complexity of compliance behaviors and providing an explanation for why simplistic interventions such as alternative pressure modes have not made a substantial impact on compliance.[115–119] A Cochrane meta-analysis of nontechnical methods to improve CPAP compliance in the general OSA population showed that supportive and educational interventions can modestly increase use and that cognitive behavioral therapies may lead to a larger increase of machine use.[69] In most studies where telemedicine was used, a cognitive behavioral intervention was applied by telephone,[6,9,75,83,84,120] the Internet,[6,75] or videoconference.[20,48,63]

Active calls and automated telephone-linked communication/digitized human speech

Demolles and colleagues[84] used a daily computer-based telephone system to monitor patients' self-reported compliance behavior and provided automated counseling through a structured dialogue. The impact of the intervention was not significant in comparison to standard care. However, the findings suggest that concurrent education and reinforcement during the initial and early treatment period are effective countermeasures to patient-reported attenuated compliance. Sparrow and colleagues[9] applied an automated telemedicine intervention system, based on an algorithmic interactive voice response system designed to improve CPAP adherence and compliance. The system monitors CPAP-related symptoms and patients' self-reported behavior and provides feedback and counseling through a structured dialogue to promote CPAP use. The monitor uses digitized human speech to speak to the patients and the patients communicate via the touch-tone keypad of their telephones. Each call began with an assessment of the self-reported duration and frequency of CPAP use during the past week, followed by one of several motivational counseling modules. If the participant reported excessive side effects or OSA symptoms, the system then recommended the patient to contact his or her physician to discuss the problems. The computer system called the patients if they did not make a call at the expected times. Routine printed reports were sent to the participants' physician biweekly during the first month and the month thereafter. It was found that this telemedicine approach resulted in a median CPAP use that was 0.9 hours per night (at 6 months) and 2.0 hours per night (at 12 months) higher than that of an attention control group.[9] Chervin and colleagues performed an RCT among 33 patients of 2 interventions to improve compliance: 1 group received weekly telephone calls to uncover any problems and encourage use, a second group received written information about OSA and the importance of CPAP adherence, and finally, a third group served as a control group. The authors reported that intervention improved CPAP compliance and that the effect was especially strong when intervention occurred during the first month of CPAP treatment.[60] Isetta and colleagues[49] found in a series of 50 consecutive patients with OSA that most of them were satisfied with the teleconsultation method, and 66% agreed that the teleconsultation could replace more than half of their CPAP follow-up visits. Finally, Coma del Corral and colleagues[29] found that the level of good CPAP compliance was 85% at 6 months in patients attending the sleep center for a face-to-face meeting, whereas it was 75% in the teleconsultation arm.

Sedhaoui and colleagues performed an RCT in 379 patients with OSA, comparing standard support completed or not within 3 months of coaching sessions, based on telephone-based counseling by competent staff. Of the patients in the standard group, 65% showed a compliance rate of greater than 3 hours per night versus 75% for the coached group. The mean CPAP use was 26 minutes longer in the coached group versus standard group.[121]

These automated interventions improved adherence in part by improving motivation, altering the perception of treatment efficacy, and affect psychological constructs that determine behavior change.

Web-based access to own positive airway pressure data

Kuna and colleagues[122] tracked website use and found in an RCT that providing patients with daily web-based access to their own PAP use improves compliance (4.7 ± 3.3 hours in the usual care group, 5.9 ± 2.5 hours, and 6.3 ± 2.5 hours in the web access groups with and without financial incentive respectively). However, only about one-half of the participants logged in during the first week, and the proportion of patients using the website decreased with time. Inclusion of a financial incentive in the first week had no additive effect in improving compliance. These findings are consistent with a similar study evaluating the effect on compliance when an interactive website providing PAP data to both patients and providers is used.[89] This website, called MyCPAP, included the following components: (1) basic education regarding OSA and CPAP, (2) patient access to their own data, (3) questionnaires to assess subjective symptoms, (4) interactive guide to learn about practical solutions to their identified CPAP problem, and (5) education regarding how to use and care for CPAP and accessories.[89] Taylor and colleagues[75] used computers to provide daily Internet-based informational support and feedback (Health Buddy, daily survey) for problems experienced during CPAP use. Questions related to CPAP use, hours of sleep and quality of sleep were sent to the participants via a computer. The patient's responses were monitored by the sleep medicine practitioner, and the patient telephoned if deemed necessary. They found no significant differences between the telemedicine intervention and standard care group at 30 days in patient functional status and satisfaction with CPAP. This intervention only provided self-reported data to the health care provider, whereas objective compliance and detailed physiologic information may have been more useful in effectively troubleshooting problems and may have improved CPAP compliance.[20,75,85] Furthermore, in a RCT, Fox and colleagues[6] demonstrated improved CPAP compliance with a web-based telemedicine monitoring system. An autoCPAP machine transmitted physiologic data (residual AHI, air leak, compliance) daily to a website that could be reviewed. In case problems were identified from data from the website, the patient was contacted by telephone as necessary.[6] After 3 months, the mean compliance rate was significantly greater in the telemedicine arm (191 min/d), compared with the usual care arm (105 minutes), but even then CPAP compliance was low. In contrast, 67 minutes of technician time was spent on the patients in the telemedicine arm compared with the standard approach.

Automated messaging (reinforcement emails or texts)

Various forms of telecommunication, which may include automated message data alerts, coaching and reinforcement emails, texts, and calls, as well as online educational and motivational support, have shown similar or increased CPAP compliance.[19] It is particularly interesting that this feedback process (sending positive or warning messages in the case of good or poor compliance, respectively) can be performed automatically, therefore minimizing health staff cost. Frasnelli and colleagues[78] used short text messages by SMS with treatment reinforcement was sent out weekly, if no phone calls were necessary. The Tele-OSA study of automated messaging associated with telemonitoring gave early improvement in CPAP adherence, but this effect gradually declined after discontinuation of automated feedback messaging.[93] The majority preferred to receive messages via email (31.7%), followed by text messaging (17.5%), and phone (2.3%), whereas 40% preferred a combination of approaches.[44] In the study of Hwang and colleagues,[44] the overall improvement in adherence with telemonitoring was substantial, but the degree of response varied between individual patients. In a prospective, open, multicenter study involving 122 patients with OSA, effectiveness and coaching costs were evaluated using U-Sleep, a web-based automated telehealth program.[7] In this study, the telehealth group received emails and/or text messages, whereas in the standard care arm, follow-up consisted of scheduled phone calls on days 1, 7, 14, and 30. Results of this study revealed that there was no statistically significant difference in CPAP compliance, CPAP efficacy or change in Epworth Sleepiness Scale scores between telehealth and standard care groups, but the trend favored the telehealth group. The coaching time required was significantly lower in the telehealth Group, making it a time-efficient option. The authors concluded that this automated telemedicine strategy needs to be continued indefinitely for sustained effect. Altogether, the use of technology-based approaches should be considered as 1 solution among a larger set of management strategies to personalize the care for individual patients. The potential impact of changing thresholds to increase message frequency or the possibility of personalizing automated messages for each patient, based specifically on what would motivate them the most, and individual goal setting have to be further explored.

Mobile device applications: Patient engagement tools

With increasing Internet access, there is a developing role for web-based patient engagement applications to assist patients in self-management of OSA. Recently, manufacturers of CPAP devices have designed and implemented such theory-driven coaching and support services, including a dashboard summarizing therapy data, troubleshooting and educational videos, and goal-focused automated e-mails/texting. These tools are described as patient engagement tools, self-management platforms or patient-facing applications, and should ideally include the following components: (1) remote electronic delivery, (2) personalized invitation, (3) interactive, (4) viewable on demand and as often as desired, and (5) concise and easy to understand.[93] These platforms operate through mobile device applications (U-Sleep and MyAir: ResMed, Australia; Sleep-Mapper later DreamMapper: Philips, Amsterdam, the Netherlands), sync automatically with the CPAP vendors software program, providing personal CPAP data in comprehensive graphs to each patients, and also incorporating CPAP troubleshooting materials. The data are transferred from the patients' CPAP to a remote database, the same platform used by sleep professionals to access a comprehensive report of CPAP treatment data to monitor patients. At the same time, all these patients have access to their personal CPAP data via a mobile device application or via a web portal.[123] These systems also use structured motivational enhancement techniques such as feedback and goal setting, to encourage use. Patients receive positive feedback by sending text messages to congratulate participants about their successful CPAP adherence. In contrast, feedback to patients with a poor night of adherence may motivate improved use on the subsequent night. These concepts are part of social cognitive theory, which considers self-efficacy as a major determinant of behavior change.[58,124,125] Strong self-efficacy beliefs are associated with the ability to withstand treatment failure and persist in efforts.[126,127] Altogether, these patient engagement tools enhance self-monitoring by providing the patient with easy-to-view reports of trends in use, AHI, and feedback about mask leak. MyAir also monitors mask off/on events in addition, and gives a summary score based on proprietary weighting of the aforementioned factors. Although MyCPAP provides troubleshooting tips and educational materials, they must be selected by the patient. In contrast, the commercial platforms serve up educational suggestions, based on the monitoring as well as suggestions for selecting intermediate goals of care, possibly better equipping patients to problem solve and to set goals.[47] As said, these applications also serve as a portal to educational videos about OSA and CPAP therapy, which facilitate patients to trouble shoot as problems arise.

Such an approach has shown benefit when delivered by health care providers in different studies (**Table 4**).[45,89,99,128,129,130]

Engleman and colleagues[131] presented a retrospective study (data from Philips) comparing CPAP use in an old-fashioned OSA cohort versus a new feature OSA cohort, including remote monitoring, device display and a patient support phone app. In the 817 included patients, the implementation of multiple telemedicine supporting tools resulted in an increase in daily CPAP use of 1.1 hours per night during the first 12 weeks of CPAP therapy. Pittard and colleagues[128] reported similar significant results with the DreamMapper. Hardy and colleagues reported that 78% of those who used SleepMapper were compliant at 90 days compared with 56% of those who did not, and they used CPAP for an average of 1.4 hours longer per night.[46] U-Sleep patients do have a better CPAP use at 3 months (83% vs 73%), but without statistical significance.[7] However, they found that fewer coaching minutes were required during the

3-month follow-up period for the U-Sleep (24 vs 58 minutes for usual care). This suggests that U-Sleep could be a cost-effective solution by potentially replacing traditional follow-up protocols without drop-off in CPAP adherence. Hostler and colleagues reported an 18% increase in nights with more than 4 hours of use, and patients in the SleepMapper Group were more than 3 times as likely to meet adherence criteria (>4 hours per night for 70% of nights), a trend that just missed statistical significance ($P = .06$). This should translate into significant improvements at the individual and population level.[99] A retrospective analysis of 1000 patients found that 77% of those who opted to engage with such a tool used CPAP for 4 hours or more per night, compared with 63% of those who opted out. A retrospective review of 15.000 patients in a database showed 78% of those who used SleepMapper were compliant at 90 days and used CPAP.[93] Similarly, a retrospective analysis of 128,037 patients found that a greater proportion of those who opted into the same patient engagement technology were compliant compared with those who did not (87.3% vs 70.4%, respectively).[130]

In a study that used data from a large German home care provider, it was shown that the use of a proactive patient management program supported by remote access to PAP therapy data significantly lowered therapy termination rate (5.4% vs 11.0%) and time to therapy termination was significantly longer (348 vs 337 days).[132] In another study, Woehrle and colleagues[129] also reported that the therapy termination rate was lower

Table 4
Patient engagement tools and compliance

	N	AHI	Patient Engagement Tool	Follow-up	Compliance Patient Engagement Tools	Compliance Usual Care	P Value
Stepnowsky et al,[89] 2013	241	36	MyCPAP	120 d	3.9 h	3.2 h	S
Pittard et al,[128] 2015	2173	N/A	DreamMapper	60 d	5 h	3.9 h	S
Hardy et al,[45] 2016	172678	N/A	DreamMapper	90 d	5 h	3.9 h	S
Hostler et al,[99] 2017	61	18–19	SleepMapper	77 d	4 h	2.7 h	S
Woehrle et al,[129] 2018	1000	N/A	myAir	180 d	5.4 h	4.2 h	S
Malhotra et al,[130] 2018	128037	N/A	myAir	90 d	5.9 h	4.9 h	S

Abbreviation: N/A, not applicable.

in the patient engagement group, with higher device use and lower leak. The AHI was equal in both groups. The addition of a patient engagement tool was associated with a significant improvement in device use in patients receiving CPAP therapy for the first time. Increases were seen in both the number of days with device use and in the hours of device use each night. Moreover, there was a significant reduction in leak in patients managed using a patient engagement approach compared with telemonitoring alone.[129] Potential explanations for this observation include better education and feedback compared with usual care. Patient engagement tools add another level to telemonitoring. Patients can get involved via shared decision-making with their health care givers and by increasing their health literacy (accessing, understanding and implementing health information). Moreover, the use of real-time feedback could help to keep patients actively engaged with their therapy, and remind and motivate them to use their device. Also, such technology facilitates the input of real-time clinical data and allows real-time responses that incorporate personalized recommendations based on the data received. Key features of patients engagement tools are (1) the patient believes that they have an important role to play in their own health care, (2) the patient is provided with the confidence and knowledge to take action, (3) the patient takes action to maintain and improve their health, and (4) the patient persists with the program even during times of stress.[129,133] Hwang and colleagues[44] demonstrated that Web-OSA education added to an automated CPAP follow-up program impacted CPAP adherence to a greater degree than either of those platforms used in isolation.

Apart from an improved adherence to PAP therapy, patient engagement tools are inexpensive, do not draw on health care resources, and show promise in improving PAP therapy for OSA.[47] Use of these platforms was associated with using PAP for significantly more hours per night (range of 0.7–1.3 hours more). In contrast, it could be that this difference has a minimal effect on symptom improvement, because the scores could be affected by coexisting conditions. Traditional telemonitoring systems require health care professional-initiated patient contact and deployment of health care resources, whereas patient engagement tools engage patients directly without placing additional burden on health care.[47] In a real-life big data study with 4.181.490 patients, those who registered to use an engagement tool consistently had better adherence (80%–85%) than those who did not (65%–70%).[134] Patient engagement tool use was associated with a greater than 2-fold increase in the probability of achieving sufficient adherence. The possibility arises that some patients may have been experienced PAP users before joining trials with patient engagement tools rather than new PAP users.[129,130] Such patients might behave differently to patient engagement tools than PAP-naïve patients. However, prior studies show that PAP use is established soon after PAP initiation, and it seems unlikely that providing feedback data and recommendations to experienced users would result in greater improvement in PAP adherence than what was observed in PAP-naïve patients.[122] Further efforts are needed to identify key features, their effect on outcomes of interest, and which patients would benefit from them most.

TELEMANAGEMENT OF COMORBIDITIES

Improved outcomes have been reported using telemedicine in conditions like diabetes mellitus, hypertension, stroke, and HIV.[113,135–138] This opens new horizons for patients with OSA and comorbidities. Obesity is the most frequent condition associated with OSA, which deserves close attention.

Appel and colleagues[139] evaluated the effectiveness of a telemedicine behavioral weight loss intervention among 415 obese patients with at least one cardiovascular risk factor for 2 years. Participants were randomized to the following groups: (1) remote weight loss support (by telephone, website, and email), (2) in-person support together with the 3 remote means of support, and (3) a control group with self-directed weight-loss management. After 2 years, the mean change in weight from baseline and percentage of participants who lost 5% or more of their initial weight was significantly greater in the remote support groups (with or without additional in-person interventions), when compared with the control group (with self-directed weight-loss management). Hence, the remote support interventions facilitated greater weight loss, and did not require in-person support. Another known comorbidity associated with OSA is diabetes, which has also been looked into with the use of telemedicine. Wang and colleagues[140] evaluated the use of U-health care, a remote platform based on an Internet interface that transmits glycemic data immediately through a glucometer. The intervention group received information about medicines, diet, and exercise through the platform, whereas the control group received conventional medical treatment without any additional intervention. After 18 months follow up, the intervention group achieved better glycemic control, improved hemoglobin A1c levels and decreased triglyceride levels.

This approach also improved patients' adherence to the medical team's instructions.

Heart failure can also be associated with OSA, and is one of the first fields where telemedicine has been applied. Bashi and colleagues[141] analyzed 19 systematic reviews of remote interventions that focused on the control of heart failure. The use of telemonitoring of physiologic parameters (heart rate, blood pressure, electrocardiogram, and weight) showed a reduction in heart failure hospitalization, all-cause hospitalization, mortality and an improvement in quality of life. However, there is a lack of evidence to support the effectiveness of interventions involving mobile phone use, videoconferences, or other devices.

Nevertheless, the application of new technologies is not suitable for all populations.[142,143] Therefore, it is mandatory to choose wisely the appropriate outcomes and patient populations for telehealth strategies.

TELEMEDICINE IN PARTICULAR POPULATIONS

It is remarkable that primarily those telemedicine concepts were able to increase use time in which the control group used the CPAP device for less than 4 hours per night. In contrast, when the control group is greater than the threshold of 4 hours per night, usually no further improvement is achieved.

A recent meta-analysis revealed that telemedicine care was associated with significantly greater CPAP compliance compared with usual care, with a pooled mean difference of 0.68 hours per night.[97] However, the findings need to be interpreted with caution, given the varying methodologic quality of the included studies, the high heterogeneity of the recruited studies, as well as the fat that the included type and intensity of both usual care and experimental interventions varied considerably. Another meta-analysis included 22 studies, and showed that telemedicine interventions are able to increase adherence to CPAP treatment.[96] However, in 10 studies no significant effect was found on compliance, although 57% of the patients were from a single center that was in favor of telemonitoring. Hence, the exact level of educational and supportive concepts in the control groups contributed to the additional effect of telemedical interventions. Probably, a ceiling effect regarding educational actions must be considered.[101] Similarly, Schoch and colleagues[8] concluded that the telemedicine intervention did not significantly improve CPAP use in an unselected OSA population, which was explained by a relatively high adherence in the control arm. In contrast, the same group found a positive impact on CPAP use in a subgroup of patients with a milder form of OSA. Also, significant improvement in quality of life was found, which was not related to the hours of CPAP use, but was most pronounced in the telemedicine arm. This brings us to a more general aspect concerning the target population, namely whether the whole CPAP-treated population should be included, or only particular phenotypes that are better served for different aspects of telehealth options.[144]

It could be argued that telemonitoring might be more useful in specific populations (eg, poorly adherent patients or those with few symptoms) and also reinforces the concept that better adherence and treatment effectiveness can only be ensured by using distinctive tailored management strategies, with or without telemonitoring, according to the OSA phenotype.[145] For patients with comorbid insomnia, telemedicine also opens opportunities to exchange and automatically process sleep diaries, smartphone applications of sleep-wake data and follow online programs related to cognitive behavioral therapy.[146–148] This way, the insomnia field can probably be transitioned from evaluating more basic, noninteractive online programs to personalized, interactive online programs. For example, the group of Espie and colleagues[147] used a virtual therapist to help deliver a web-based cognitive behavioral therapy-i program. Such approach may likely have more important roles in managing insomnia in the future. Apart from insomnia, it has been shown that the cognitive behavioral therapy approach is also effective in a context of OSA to improve CPAP adherence.[149] In case of inadequate sleep hygiene, platforms can be programmed with automated messages to encourage behavioral change, without direct interaction with the sleep provider.[150]

One major limitation in telemonitoring studies is the failure to reach a sufficient sample size. In a recent French study it was found that 1646 patients would have been needed to reach a power of 0.8 to show a significant difference of 0.34 hour per night in compliance, whereas 788 patients would have been needed to meet a threshold of greater than 0.5 hours with a power of 0.80.[104] This may also suggest that it is unlikely that a meaningful increase in CPAP adherence of less than 30 minutes is clinically significant.

Hence, the American Academy of Sleep Medicine guideline recommends telemonitoring-guided interventions during the initial period of PAP therapy in adults with OSA, but only at conditional level of recommendation.[53,54] It seems that a wise balance between enthusiasm and skepticism, which is inherently linked with solid science, would be the best way to consolidate useful results for routine application of telemedicine for

PAP follow-up in OSA. The field is at a very early stage for pediatric patients compared with adult ones, and no systematic reviews have been carried out on telemedicine for pediatric OSA. So, it is unclear whether the results could be generalized to younger populations. Finally, in stroke patients, Kotzian and colleagues[100] reported a higher compliance in telemonitored patients after 3 months, after 1 year there was no significant difference. Nilius and colleagues[101] studied stroke patients as well and found a higher compliance after 6 months of home therapy.

PATIENT SATISFACTION

There are a multitude of potential benefits to incorporating telemedicine into adult sleep practices, including and not limited to saving travel time and costs, less missed work time, and eventually bringing multiple caregivers together. Smartphones allow almost all health care professionals to connect seamlessly and attend telemedicine appointments. Such approach may also decrease appointment no-show rates. Surprisingly, in the study of Turino and colleagues telemonitoring system was unexpectedly associated with lower patient satisfaction. The study observed no significant difference in neither percentage of patients with good adherence nor 3-month use hour per night between the 2 groups. This finding was explained by the lack of in-person contact in the intervention arm, whereas clinical appointments were only scheduled for the control arm.[80] Also, in the study of Bros and colleagues,[151] a majority (78%) of patients expressed a favorable attitude toward telemonitoring, but nearly 40% considered the telemonitoring device like intrusive. Telemonitoring also encompasses the risk to mask some aspects of care, by relying excessively on technical parameters, forgetting the clinical context.[21] This could result in a decrease in medical quality and dehumanization of care, missing the fact that monitoring CPAP use can be satisfying, but in a patient suffering from residual excessive daytime sleepiness, it is not the complete picture.[67] Whereas dehumanization of care with telemonitoring is a significant concern for the physician–patient relationship, this parallel route should not be underestimated. Moreover, it is very unlikely that telemedicine will completely replace face-to-face contacts. Importantly, the perfect match of both routes (with and without in-person visits) will likely improve health care as a whole.[152]

ECONOMIC APPROACH

Cost effectiveness is an important factor to consider when discussing the role of telemedicine in OSA, keeping in mind the ever-increasing health care expenses. Telemedicine can contribute to the improved cost effectiveness of OSA management during both the diagnostic and therapeutic phases. However, we must be cautious when applying these methods to the clinical setting, given that some studies have described that the intervention could not always be cost effective or even could induce negative outcomes. The evidence for unequivocally positive outcomes on patient health is still limited. Costs mostly depend on staff time and hardware expenses. Nevertheless, in a simulation of the cost effect, it was shown that if half of the patients were managed by telemedicine, the nationwide annual cost for management of patients with OSA would decrease with 17%.[105]

Staff Time

Telemonitoring could be a time- and human resource-intensive tool for sleep centers and homecare providers. Frequent involvement of staff through in-person contacts or automated feedback triggering may counteract cost-effectiveness, because the same effects might be achieved through routine phone calls without the use of telemedicine device.[8] Reviewing the downloaded information every week day is labor intensive and may not be feasible in all settings. One misunderstanding could be that patients consider their physicians to be routinely monitoring their data on a regular basis. However, such expectations cannot be met without having intermediary support (such as respiratory therapists or home-care providers) to assign certain trigger thresholds for the PAP compliance data to trigger when compliance is not being met.[39] Fox and colleagues[6] quantified provider time and found that an additional 67 minutes on overage per patient was spent managing the patients that were remotely monitored. A much greater number of interventions can be expected in the telemonitored patients. In patients with OSA with at least 1 intervention, an overall 59% increase in the number of physician interventions and 54% increase in the number of homecare provider's interventions was shown.[104] This finding emphasizes the need for a cost-effectiveness validation of such a strategy, given the greater burden of caregivers' interventions for both medical (persistent high residual AHI, residual sleepiness) and technical (masks, humidifiers) reasons. It could be speculated that a usual care intervention might be more efficient from a cost perspective, given that an average of 30 minutes may be necessary to respond to or to manage each alert.[104] In contrast, multimedia approaches could also help save nursing time, which could inherently allow more patients to be managed with the same manpower.[7,98] Recent studies demonstrated a reduction in labor requirements, nursing time and cost owing to telemedical care.[7,80,98] Office staff telemonitoring of voluminous nightly data from entire practices of patients is daunting and generally not reimbursable. However, telemedicine may provide a pragmatic solution for practices attempting to manage huge amounts of nightly CPAP data for PAP patients over years. It is also not clear how long special patient groups, like people who had a stroke, might benefit from telemedicine while treated with PAP. In stroke patients, the costs seemed to be low, since the use increase was achieved with an average of 4.7 contacts per patient over a period of 6 months.[101] The telemedicine concept led to a reduction of daytime sleepiness and blood pressure and might help increase quality of life after the stroke. Thanks to targeting of interventions to patients with problems observed, one can focus precious working hours on those PAP patients who really need additional support.

Equipment

Furthermore, telemedicine is rather expensive, and this is related to the complex technology required to implement telecare. These costs could be decreased by wider use of telemedicine in the future. As discussed earlier, Coma-del-Corral and colleagues[29] investigated telemonitored polygraphy in patients with clinical suspicion of OSAS. Telemedicine-polygraphy was performed on 40 patients, in a virtual sleep unit, in another hospital some 80 km from the central sleep laboratory. The sleep laboratory nurses performed real-time continuous telemedicine-polygraphy check. Continuous video monitoring (via a webcam) was also available. No polygraphy failure was observed, but data transmission failed for 2.5% of the recordings. The cost analysis showed also that telemedicine is associated with additional costs: telemedicine-polygraphy cost 277 € compared with 145 € for a PSG.[29,153]

Access to health care

Another interesting aspect is that telemedicine can improve the efficiency of health care delivery in terms of costs and time. Of course, when setting up a telemedicine visit, the patients should be reassured that they will still receive the same level of care as they would get face to face. Studies reported a decrease in travel costs and office room rentals, which will likely not apply in all countries, because economic times and public transportation policies strongly differ. Russo and colleagues[154] analyzed the savings associated with

a telemedicine program conducted between 2005 and 2013. This program was associated with average travel savings of 145 miles and 142 minutes per visit, and access to health care services was streamlined and made more convenient for patients. Other wider benefits include decreased fuel consumption and carbon emissions associated with traveling to a clinical review. It is clear that these cost savings are most substantial for individuals in rural areas or areas without a sleep clinic.[20] Surprisingly, the use of supporting tools generally results in better adherence, although it is not effective to change lifestyle and behaviors.[102] Furthermore, the application of advanced devices depends largely on individual income, and thus is not useful for most patients of lower socioeconomic status.[97] A few studies were conducted among Asian patients with OSA. Murase and colleagues[105] showed the noninferiority of a telemonitoring system at 3-month follow-up in CPAP adherence, whereas Chumpangern and colleagues[79,155,156] reported an insignificantly higher CPAP compliance, and adherence was significantly higher in the telemonitoring group.

More Efficient Management of Resources: Addition of Artificial Intelligence

Telemedicine and Internet of things provide unprecedented opportunities for integrating comanagement approaches, multi-actor interactions and patient empowerment, and will generate a data deluge that could be addressed by advanced analytics.[39] Integrating information from diagnostic testing and positive airway pressure compliance databases could allow providers and systems to more efficiently manage resources. As an example, artificial intelligence could phenotype certain patient groups based on demographics or comorbidities and help providers allocate resources to those patients who have more complex diseases while providing lower cost care to patients who are doing well and unlikely to benefit from the more resource intensive model of care.[157] Instead of managing all patients in a similar fashion, data-driven decision-making could allow providers to better allocate resources, maintain or improve quality, reduce the cost of care, and improve value for insurers, providers, and patients.[157] In such a model, coordination of care with improved quality and efficiency will be valued more than the quantity of care that currently drives the traditional fee-for-service system.

Reimbursement

The promise of expanded OSA telemedicine applications is accompanied with cautious considerations. Practical implementation into clinical OSA workflows requires an understanding of local payment for teleservices as well as assessment of available resources.

Practices may want to project potential lost in-person clinic revenue during telemedicine clinics and balance potential financial gains, because telemedicine visits may not be reimbursed at parity with in-person visits. Reimbursement at a relevant level for services rendered is the cornerstone of long-term revenue. Nevertheless, telemonitoring-guided support for PAP-treated patients reduces the number of patients terminating therapy, can improve PAP use, reduce the workload associated with follow-up for care providers, and will improve the economic model of treating sleep apnea patients at the end.[129]

Need for Cost–Benefit Studies

Further studies are needed to clarify if personalized concepts with telemonitoring and direct patient contact or fully automated feedback messaging systems are more cost effective and achieve similar adherence results.[101] The likelihood of improved adherence with telemedicine interventions will need to be balanced against the resources needed to implement the program and will require robust cost effectiveness evaluations. Well-designed and adequately powered trials are needed to establish whether this approach is a clinically effective and cost-effective option for CPAP management. Future studies could specifically adopt both societal and health care perspectives in examining cost effectiveness in comparison with usual care.

CHANGING PARADIGMS AND EXPANDING HORIZONS

Based on evidence from the literature discussed in this article, outcomes seem to favor telemedicine approaches. The evolution of sleep medicine care is full of incredible opportunities given its natural reliance of technology and relevance to so many medical specialties.[39] The potential for telemedicine to change and restructure current care management paradigms is immense. Telemedicine can provide the links between sleep specialists, primary care, industry, and the multidisciplinary sleep team.

Management Outside the Office

Evidence supports the noninferiority of synchronous telemonitoring compared with usual care for adherence. Using a combination of face-to-face telemedicine appointments, cloud-based positive airway pressure compliance monitoring,

and Internet-based communications and coaching, it is likely that many patients with uncomplicated OSA could be managed successfully outside of the office setting.[7,44,76] For those patients who are doing well with their positive airway pressure therapy (or other treatments), a simple tele-health visit or Internet-based communication could suffice, leaving more time for patients with more complex problems to be evaluated in an office setting.[158] Also, self-monitoring of blood pressure and weight is gaining interest. Mendelson and colleagues[159] showed the feasibility of patient entry of blood pressure, CPAP use, sleepiness and quality of life data for clinician review, and McManus and colleagues[160] reported that patient self-monitoring of blood pressure, with or without telemonitoring, decreased blood pressure values after 1 year. These trends will certainly modify the patient–physician relationships.

Monitoring of Therapies Other Than Continuous Positive Airway Pressure

Emerging technologies are available that have sleep (position) e-monitoring capabilities.[161] For instance, telemonitoring of oral appliance compliance data is feasible, based on temperature-sensing data chips embedded in the oral appliance. When combining with triple axis accelerometer technologies, oral appliance use times as well as supine versus nonsupine data can be monitored, and eventually shared web based between patient and care giver.[161] Similar developments take place for hypoglossal nerve stimulation devices.[162]

Lifestyle Modification

Telemonitoring of CPAP devices is now proposed as one component of a more complex and integrated strategy that use mobile health applications and wearable sensors to monitor physiologic parameters, such as blood pressure, body weight, sleep duration, and physical activity. This also emphasizes the changing perspective regarding sleep, as it is currently considered at least as important as exercise or diet in general health.[163] As stated elsewhere in this article, regarding comorbidities, CPAP treatment supported by a telemedicine system that included monitoring of blood pressure and sent reminders for physical activity and healthy diet via smartphones did not demonstrate efficacy in reducing cardiovascular risk in patients with OSA when used as secondary prevention.[159]

In another study, telemonitoring was not superior to usual CPAP care for improving home blood pressure in patients with OSA and high cardiovascular risk.[102] CPAP compliance was 0.53 hours higher compared with usual care, which was statistically significant, but the modest difference in CPAP adherence between the 2 arms was probably not enough to induce a significant reduction in blood pressure. In contrast, total cholesterol and triglyceride levels were significantly lowered, and high-density lipoprotein cholesterol improved in the telemonitoring arm. Also, patient-centered outcomes, namely, sleepiness and quality of life, improved. In symptomatic patients with OSA with low cardiovascular risk, the implementation of multimodal telemonitoring did not give better CPAP adherence than usual care. The success of telemonitoring may be dependent on knowing who best responds to these new telemedicine approaches (age, education, geographic setting, race, phenotype, cluster).

Expanding Applications of Smartphone Apps and Wearables

Sleep apps remain among the most popular apps downloaded for Apple and Android devices.[164] The number of apps is continuously growing, and a multitude of them claim to track and define sleep-related metrics, improve sleep quality, and even screen for sleep disorders. Unfortunately, these apps lack minimal validation regarding the ability to accurately perform these functions. Equally, consumer sleep technologies (wearables) are self-described lifestyle/entertainment devices that are not subject to US Food and Drug Administration approval. Although patients may not be as concerned about this lack of validation, they seem to recognize some shortcomings of consumer health-related technology. At the best, these apps and wearables could be considered in the context of a comprehensive sleep evaluation, but should not replace validated diagnostic instruments. Also, minimal validation data exist regarding the ability of consumer sleep technologies to perform the functions that they purport to. However, these devices become increasingly sophisticated, some may undergo validation and ultimately have a role in clinical care. So, it is important to acknowledge them as adjuncts that may help with communication with patients, goal setting, and increasing patient engagement.[165] Even more, by making use of environmental factors, like ambient light, ambient noise, accelerometer analysis to detect nonmovement patterns, and smartphone use patterns allows clinicians to accurately estimate the owner's wake and sleep behavior. One promising approach is to add low-cost oximetry probes to a smartphone. Given the need of a continuous oximetry curve over a full night, this would put additional demands on the

system in terms of battery power. Also, beat-to-beat processing is important to maintain the rapid changes in oximetry, which are very typical for sleep apnea and not observed in other conditions.[4] Apps could also be helpful to empower patients. Isetta and colleagues developed an mHealth app called APPnea, aimed at promoting patients self-monitoring of CPAP treatment. APPnea gave patients daily reminders to answer 3 questions about their OSA treatment ("Did you use your CPAP more than 4 hour last night? Did you perform any physical activity yesterday? Did you follow the dietary advice given? and once weekly the app prompted the user to answer "How much do you weigh?"). Those patients who used APPnea regularly showed a trend toward higher CPAP compliance (+0.5 hours per night).[166] The world of wearables and apps is here to stay, and our job is to figure out how to unlock the unlimited possibilities. Integration of these wearable sensors may add further actionable data that can potentially facilitate disease management.

Integration in the e-Health Sleep Record

Ideally, the data from CPAP devices should to be incorporated with the data regarding the physical status of the patients into the e-health sleep record. In a later stage, other aspects of digital technology will most likely be incorporated. Among them, integration of relevant health-related data collected from everyday apparel, wearable sensors and household appliances, increased interactivity between patients and health care provider, anticipation, and thus, hopefully prevent, worsening of medical disease states based on validated algorithms. Moreover, some consumer sleep technologies, usually smartphone- or tablet-based, to track or modify sleep are becoming widely available.[167] These applications are transitioning to reliably track snoring, sleep, oximetry, heart rate and presence of sleep apnea. At the same time, artificial intelligence algorithms and software to collect individual and group analysis of body weight, blood pressure, sleepiness, and other data for prediction models are advancing. Pathways need to be explored for special populations or patients with combination sleep, breathing, medical, or comorbid disorders. How to best incorporate these and other new entities into best-practice standard, hybrid, and telemedicine OSA workflows currently seems a moving average.

Remaining Barriers in the Incorporation of Telemedicine into Routine Clinical Practice

Generalization of the use of telemedicine has been hampered by multiple practical barriers, such as the use of different CPAP brands, the lack of standardization of parameters used by different providers, preventing interoperability for health care professionals and the management of data within the existing electronic patient files.[123] Some concerns could be raised because of the limitation to perform a physical examination during teleconsultations. However, some elements of the examination, such as blood pressure or body weight can be easily obtained by the nurse or primary care physician.[123] Moreover, elderly subjects, who may benefit most from telemedicine services, may be disadvantaged because of cultural and practical barriers.[168] Similarly, economic issues may prevent use of telemedicine services in subjects with low socioeconomic status. From a data safety and health care regulation point of view, there is ongoing discussion about which data have to be regarded as general wellness and lifestyle data and which data have to be regarded as health care data to be used for medical diagnostic purposes.[4] Many regulatory aspects are still open to this kind of application. Also, reimbursement issues remain.

COVID-19: Changing the Interest in Telemedicine

Since the start of the lockdown for COVID-19, the clinical activity regarding patients with sleep-disordered breathing has stopped owing to the limited access of patients to the hospital, and the risk of droplet dispersion associated with the use of ©PAP.[169] According to a multicenter European study, a minority of sleep centers used telemedicine regularly during the first COVID-19 lockdown, mostly to monitor compliance to treatment rather than for full clinical management.[170] Care for patients with OSA is a highly specialized, because they are often aged and have multiple comorbidities.[171] The high prevalence of OSA in the general population is associated with long waiting lists, further lengthened during the pandemic. Telemedicine could potentially tackle this problem,[21,123] but has not been included yet among the services provided by many health care systems.[169] A paradigm shift in sleep medicine practice after the COVID-19 pandemic has been foreseen, not only for OSA, but also for other sleep problems.[172] Last year, interest in telemedicine for the management of patients with OSA is emerging, with identification of advantages and drawbacks.[173] Studies have mostly addressed questions regarding the role of telemedicine in monitoring compliance to CPAP treatment, or follow-up after the initiation of treatment for OSA, but overall advantages over usual care were small, as the results of telemedicine care were comparable to, and costs were slightly lower than the usual sleep laboratory-centered management.[50] The COVID-19 pandemic has dramatically raised the issue of safety, changing the balance in favor of telemedicine, and will likely grow in the future. COVID-19 has also accelerated efforts to regulate but also to bill telehealth care, which will fasten the implementation of telemedicine.

SUMMARY

In this review, we demonstrated that telemedicine applications can be useful to monitor and motivate sleep apnea patients on a large scale. However, the effect sizes for compliance for telemedicine approaches are not as large as what has been achieved with the use of theory-driven approaches such as cognitive behavioral therapy, and the impacts on patient and provider satisfaction and cost effectiveness are not yet clear. These aspects of OSA care do not require substantial changes in care programs and strategies. In contrast, remotely monitored sleep studies and CPAP titration require more resources together with a change in patient care management. Given the turning hospital strategies toward more ambulatory care, telemedicine is going to evolve and it is very likely that there will be an increasing development of tools and activities in all areas of sleep medicine. Currently, efforts are being made to regulate but also to bill telehealth care, which will accelerate the implementation of telemedicine. This will certainly change the daily clinical practice, but we have to take into account the limitations of these techniques.

In future, large-scale adequately powered pragmatic clinical trials are needed to better understand the effectiveness and the role of the telemedicine approach in managing sleep-disordered breathing. Evidence for the long-term follow-up effectiveness of telemonitoring interventions in improving adherence to CPAP treatment remains undecided owing to a scarcity of available studies and their mixed results. What happens when patients are no longer monitored or followed-up by visits to the clinic after their first months using the CPAP machine? Challenges and growing pains are to be expected, but clinical needs, existing technology, and opportunities for growth abound.

CLINICS CARE POINTS

- Careful telemedicine management will provide a more seamless communication flow, to the benefit of medical providers, the global health care system, and ultimately for patients.
- Telemedicine ensures communication during the pandemic despite environmental barriers.
- Telemedicine can facilitate access to sleep medicine, and is not necessarily limited to rural areas.
- Use of filters is mandatory in order not to be overloaded by a tsunami of data.
- Advantages of telemedicine have to be weighed versus the resources required to offer qualitative telemedicine care.
- Although synchronous telemonitoring is noninferior compared to usual care, ceiling effects regarding compliance play a role if the standard care is already of high quality.
- The success of telemonitoring may be dependent on knowing who best responds to these new telemedicine approaches (age, education, geographic setting, race, phenotype, cluster, patients with certain conditions), and special considerations could be necessary in specific target groups.

DISCLOSURE

Dr. Verbraecken reports grants and personal fees from ResMed, Philips, Sanofi, Agfa-Gevaert, Bioprojet, Jazz Pharmaceutics, AirLiquide, Springer, Westfalen Medical, SomnoMed, Vivisol, Total Care, Medidis, Fisher & Paykel, Wave Medical, OSG, Mediq Tefa, NightBalance, Heinen & Löwenstein, AstraZen,Accuramed, Bekaert Deslee Academy, UCB Pharma, Desitin, Idorsia, and Inspire Medical Systems, all outside the submitted work..

REFERENCES

1. Freedman N. Counterpoint: does laboratory polysomnography yield better outcomes than home sleep testing? No. Chest 2015;148(2):308–10.
2. Parish J, Freedman N, Manaker S. Evolution in reimbursement for sleep studies and sleep centers. Chest 2015;147(3):600–6.
3. Venkateshiah SB, Hoque R, Collop NA. Legal aspects of sleep medicine in the 21th Century. Chest 2018;154(3):691–8.
4. Penzel T, Schöbel C, Fietze I. New technology to assess sleep apnea: wearables, smartphones, and accessories. F1000Res 2018;7:413.
5. Singh J, Badr MS, Diebert W, et al. American Academy of Sleep Medicine (AASM) Position paper for the use of telemedicine for the diagnosis and treatment of sleep disorders. J Clin Sleep Med 2015; 11(10):1187–98.
6. Fox N, Hirsch-Allen AJ, Goodfellow E, et al. The impact of telemedicine monitoring system on positive airway pressure adherence in patients with obstructive sleep apnea: a randomized controlled trial. Sleep 2012;35(4):477–81.
7. Munafo D, Hevener W, Crocker M, et al. A telehealth program for CPAP adherence reduces labor and yields similar adherence and efficacity when compared to standard of care. Sleep Breath 2016;20:777–85.
8. Schoch OD, Baty F, Boesch M, et al. Telemedicine for continuous positive airway pressure in sleep apnea. A randomized, controlled study. Ann Am Thorac Soc 2019;16(12):1550–7.
9. Sparrow D, Aloia M, Demolles DA, et al. A telemedicine intervention to improve adherence to continuous positive airway pressure: a randomised controlled trial. Thorax 2010;65:1061–6.
10. Stepnowsky CJ Jr, Palau JJ, Marler MR, et al. Pilot randomized trial of the effect of wireless telemonitoring on compliance and treatment efficacy in obstructive sleep apnea. J Med Internet Res 2007;9(2):e14.
11. Aurora RN, Quan SF. Quality measure for screening for adult obstructive sleep apnea by primary care physicians. J Clin Sleep Med 2016;12(8):1185–7.
12. Chai-Coetzer CL, Antic NA, Rowland LS, et al. Primary care vs specialist sleep center management of obstructive sleep apnea and daytime sleepiness and quality of life: a randomized trial. JAMA 2013; 309(10):997–1004.
13. Kapur VK, Auckley DH, Chowdhuri S, et al. Clinical practice guideline for diagnostic testing for adult obstructive sleep apnea: an American Academy of Sleep Medicine Clinical Practice Guideline. J Clin Sleep Med 2017;13:479–504.
14. Chang Y, Staley B, Simonsen S, et al. Transitioning from paper to electronic health record collection of Epworth sleepiness scale (ESS) for quality measures. Sleep 2018;41(1):404.
15. Stretch R, Ryden A, Fung CH, et al. Predicting nondiagnostic home sleep apnea tests using machine learning. J Clin Sleep Med 2019;15(11):1599–608.
16. Sunwoo BY, Light M, Malhotra A. Strategies to augment adherence in the management of sleep-disordered breathing. Respirology 2020;25(4): 363–71.
17. Mencar C, Gallo C, Mantero, et al. Application of machine learning to predict obstructive sleep apnea syndrome (OSAS) severity. Health Inform J 2019;26(1):298–317.

18. Budhiraja R, Thomas R, Kim M, et al. The role of big data in the management of sleep-disordered breathing. Sleep Med Clin 2016;11:241–55.

19. Schutte-Rodin S. Telehealth, telemedicine, and obstructive sleep apnea. Sleep Med Clin 2020; 15(3):359–75.

20. Spaulding R, Stevens D, Velasquez SE. Experience with telehealth for sleep monitoring and sleep laboratory management. J Telemed Telecare 2011; 17(7):346–9.

21. Bruyneel M. Telemedicine in the diagnosis and treatment of sleep apnoea. Eur Respir Rev 2019; 28(151):180093.

22. Pelletier-Fleury N, Lanoé JL, Philippe C, et al. Economic studies and 'technical' evaluation of telemedicine: the case of telemonitored polysomnography. Health Policy 1999;49:179–94.

23. Gagnadoux F, Pelletier-Fleury N, Philippe C, et al. Home unattended vs hospital telemonitored polysomnography in suspected obstructive sleep apnea syndrome: a randomized crossover trial. Chest 2002;121(3):753–8.

24. Kristo DA, Eliasson AH, Poropatich RK, et al. Telemedicine in the sleep laboratory: feasibility and economic advantages of polysomnograms transferred online. Telemed J E Health 2001;7:219–24.

25. Kayyali HA, Weimer S, Frederick C, et al. Remotely attended home monitoring of sleep disorders. Telemed J E Health 2008;14:371–4.

26. Bruyneel M, Sanida C, Art G, et al. Sleep efficiency during sleep studies: results of a prospective study comparing home-based and in-hospital based polysomnography. J Sleep Res 2011;20:201–6.

27. Bruyneel M, Van den Broecke S, Libert W, et al. Real-time attended home-polysomnography with telematic data transmission. Int J Med Inform 2013;82(8):696–701.

28. Pelletier-Fleury N, Gagnadoux F, Philippe C, et al. A cost-minimization study of telemedicine. Int J Technol Assess Health Care 2001;17(4):604–11.

29. Coma-del-Corral MJ, Alonso-Alvarez ML, Allende M, et al. Reliability of telemedicine in the diagnosis and treatment of sleep apnea Syndrome. Telemed J E Health 2013;19(1):7–12.

30. Masa JF, Corral J, Pereira R, et al. Effectiveness of home respiratory polygraphy for the diagnosis of sleep apnoea and hypopnoea syndrome. Thorax 2011;66:567–73.

31. Borsini E, Blanco M, Bosio M, et al. "Diagnosis of sleep apnea in network" respiratory polygraphy as a decentralization strategy. Sleep Sci 2016;9: 244–8.

32. Fields BG, Behari PP, McCloskey S, et al. Remote ambulatory management of veterans with obstructive sleep apnea. Sleep 2016;39(3):501–9.

33. Seo J, Choi J, Choi b, et al. The development of a nonintrusive home-based physiologic signal measurement system. Telemed J E Health 2005; 11:487–95.

34. Choi JM, Choi BH, Seo JW, et al. A system for ubiquitous health monitoring in the bedroom via a Bluetooth network and wireless LAN. Engineering in Medicine and Biology Society 2004. EMBC 2004, conference proceedings. 26th Annual International Conference of the IEEE, 2004;2: 3362-3365. San Francisco, September 1-5, 2004.

35. Boehning N, Zucchini W, Hörstmeier O, et al. Sensitivity and specificity of telemedicine-based long-term pulse-oximetry in comparison with cardiorespiratory polygraphy and polysomnography in patients with obstructive sleep apnoea syndrome. J Telemed Telecare 2011;17:15–9.

36. Boehning N, Blau A, Kujumdshieva B, et al. Preliminary results from a telemedicine referral network for early diagnosis of sleep apnoea in sleep laboratories. J Telemed Telecare 2009;15(4):203–7.

37. American Academy of sleep medicine clinical resources for #SleepTechnology. Available at: https://aasm.org/consumer-clinical-sleep-technology/. Accessed April 5, 2021.

38. Penzel T. Sleep quality challenges and opportunities. Piscataway: IEEE EMB Pulse; 2016.

39. Pepin JL, Tamisier R, Hwang D, et al. Does remote monitoring change OSA management and CPAP adherence? Respirology 2017;22(8):1508–17.

40. Nadeem R, Rishi MA, Srinivasan L, et al. Effect of visualization of raw graphic polysomnography data by sleep apnea patients on adherence to CPAP therapy. Respir Care 2013;58(4):607–13.

41. Jurado-Gamez B, Bardwell WA, Cordova-Pacheco LJ, et al. A basic intervention improves CPAP adherence in sleep apnoea patients: a controlled trial. Sleep Breath 2015;19(2):509–14.

42. Falcone VA, Damiani MF, Quaranta VN, et al. Polysomnograph chart view by patients: a new educational strategy to improve CPAP adherence in sleep apnea therapy. Respir Care 2014;59(2):193–8.

43. Rowland S, Aiyappan V, Hennessy C, et al. Comparing the efficacy, mask leak, patient adherence, and patient preference of three different CPAP interfaces to treat moderate-severe obstructive sleep apnea. J Clin Sleep Med 2018;14(1): 101–8.

44. Hwang D, Chang JW, Benjafield AV, et al. Effect of telemedicine education and telemonitoring on continuous positive airway pressure adherence. The Tele-OSA randomized trial. Am J Respir Crit Care Med 2018;197(1):117–26.

45. Hardy W, Powers J, Jasko JG, et al. DreamMapper white paper: a mobile application and website to engage sleep apnea patients in PAP therapy and improve adherence to treatment. Available at: http://incenter.medical.philips.com/doclib/enc/fetch/2000/4504/577242/577256/588723/588747/

sleepmappertx-whitepaper.pdf%3fnodeid%3d11
228847%26vernum%3d-2. Accessed April 5,
2021.

46. Lynch S, Blasé A, Erikli L, et al. Retrospective
descriptive study of CPAP adherence associated with
use of the ResMed myAir application. ResMed; 2015.
Available at: https://pdfs.semanticscholar.org/bc8e/
2341489e89cf76eeae0e76aaccb82a091c92.pdf.
Accessed April 5, 2021.

47. Shaughnessy GF, Morgenthaler TI. The effect of
patient-facing applications on positive airway pressure therapy adherence: a systematic review.
J Clin Sleep Med 2019;15(5):769–77.

48. Smith CE, Dauz ER, Clements F, et al. Telehealth
services to improve nonadherence: a placebo-
controlled study. Telemed J E Health 2006;12(3):
289–96.

49. Isetta V, Leon C, Torres M, et al. Telemedicine-
based approach for obstructive sleep apnea management: building evidence. Interact J Med Res
2014;3:e6.

50. Isetta V, Negrin MA, Monasterio C, et al. A Bayesian
cost-effectiveness analysis of a telemedicine-based
strategy for the management of sleep apnoea: a
multicentre randomised controlled trial. Thorax
2015;70:1054–61.

51. Dellaca R, Montserrat JM, Govoni L, et al. Telemetric CPAP titration at home in patients with sleep
apnea-hypopnea syndrome. Sleep Med 2011;12:
153–7.

52. Morgenthaler TI. Practice parameters for the use of
autotitrating continuous positive airway pressure
devices for titrating pressures and treating adult
patients with obstructive sleep apnea syndrome:
an update for 2007. Sleep 2008;31:141–7.

53. Patil SP, Ayappa IA, Caples SM, et al. Treatment of
adult obstructive sleep apnea with positive airway
pressure: an American Academy of Sleep Medicine
Systematic review, meta-Analysis, and GRADE
assessment. J Clin Sleep Med 2019;15(2):301–34.

54. Patil SP, Ayappa IA, Caples SM, et al. Treatment of
adult obstructive sleep apnea with positive airway
pressure: an American Academy of Sleep Medicine clinical practice guideline. J Clin Sleep Med
2019;15(2):335–43.

55. Collard Ph, Pieters Th, Aubert G, et al. Compliance
with nasal CPAP in obstructive sleep apnea patients. Sleep Med Rev 1997;1(1):33–44.

56. Engleman HM, Wild MR. Improving CPAP use by
patients with the sleep apnoea/hypopnoea syndrome (SAHS). Sleep Med Rev 2003;7(1):81–99.

57. Pépin JL, Krieger J, Rodenstein D, et al. Effective
compliance during the first 3 months of continuous
positive airway pressure. A European prospective
study of 121 patients. Am J Respir Crit Care Med
1999;160(4):1124–9.

58. Aloia MS, Arnedt JT, Stanchina M, et al. How early
in treatment is PAP adherence established ? Revisiting night-to-night variability. Behav Sleep Med
2007;5:229–40.

59. Weaver TE, Kribbs NB, Pack AI, et al. Night to night
variability in CPAP use over first three months of
treatment. Sleep 1997;20:278–83.

60. Chervin RD, Theut S, Bassetti C, et al. Compliance
with nasal CPAP can be improved by simple interventions. Sleep 1997;20:284–9.

61. Meurice JC. Improving compliance to CPAP in
sleep apnea syndrome: from coaching to telemedicine. Rev Mal Respir 2012;29:7–10.

62. Nannapaneni S, Morgenthaler TI, Ramar K. Assessing and predicting the likelihood of interventions during routine annual follow-up visits for
management of obstructive sleep. J Clin Sleep
Med 2014;10(8):919–24.

63. Parikh R, Touvelle MN, Wang H, et al. Sleep telemedicine: patient satisfaction and treatment adherence. Telemed J E Health 2011;17(8):609–14.

64. Weaver TE, Maislin G, Dinges DF, et al. Relationship between hours of CPAP use and achieving
normal levels of sleepiness and daily functioning.
Sleep 2007;30(6):711–9.

65. Rotenberg BW, Murariu D, Pang KP. Trends in
CPAP adherence over twenty years of data collec-
tion: a flattened curve. J Otolaryngol Head Neck
Surg 2016;45(1):43.

66. Barbe F, Duran-Cantolla J, Capote F, et al. Long-
term effect of continuous positive airway pressure
in hypertensive patients with sleep apnea. Am J
Respir Crit Care Med 2010;181:718–26.

67. Gasa M, Tamisier R, Launois SH, et al. Residual
sleepiness in sleep apnea patients treated by
continuous positive airway pressure. J Sleep Res
2013;22:389–97.

68. Bouloukaki I, Giannadaki K, Mermigkis C, et al.
Intensive versus standard follow-up to improve
continuous positive airway pressure compliance.
Eur Respir J 2014;44:1262–74.

69. Wozniak DR, Lasserson TJ, Smith I. Educational,
supportive and behavioural interventions to
improve usage of continuous positive airway pressure machines in adults with obstructive sleep
apnoea. Cochrane Database Syst Rev 2014;1:
CD007736.

70. Haentjens P, Van Meerhaeghe A, Moscariello A,
et al. The impact of continuous positive airway pressure on blood pressure in patients with obstructive
sleep apnea syndrome: evidence from a meta-
analysis of placebo-controlled randomized trials.
Arch Intern Med 2007;167(8):757–64.

71. Bratton DJ, Gaisl T, Wons AM, et al. CPAP vs
mandibular advancement devices and blood pressure in patients with obstructive sleep apnea: a

systematic review and meta-analysis. JAMA 2015; 314(21):2280–93.

72. Bianchi MT, Alameddine Y, Mojica J. Apnea burden: efficacy versus effectiveness in patients using positive airway pressure. Sleep Med 2014; 15(12):1579–81.

73. Bradley TD, Logan AG, Kimoff RJ, et al. Continuous positive airway pressure for central sleep apnea and heart failure. N Engl J Med 2005;353(19): 2025–33.

74. McEvoy RD, Antic NA, Heeley E, et al. CPAP for prevention of cardiovascular events in obstructive sleep apnea. N Engl J Med 2016;375(10):919–31.

75. Taylor Y, Eliasson A, Andrada T, et al. The role of telemedicine in CPAP compliance for patients with obstructive sleep apnea syndrome. Sleep Breath 2006;10(3):132–8.

76. Hoet F, Libert W, Sanida C, et al. Telemonitoring in continuous positive airway pressuretreated patients improves delay to first intervention and early compliance: a randomized trial. Sleep Med 2017; 39:77–83.

77. Leger D, Elbaz M, Piednoir B, et al. Evaluation of the add-on NOWAPI(R) medical device for remote monitoring of compliance to continuous positive airway pressure and treatment efficacy in obstructive sleep apnea. Biomed Eng Online 2016;15:26.

78. Frasnelli M, Baty F, Niederman, et al. Effect of telemetric monitoring in the first 30 days of continuous positive airway pressure adaptation for obstructive sleep apnoea syndrome—a controlled pilot study. J Telemed Telecare 2016;22:209–14.

79. Chumpangern W, Muntham D, Chirakalwasan N. Efficacy of a telemonitoring system in continuous positive airway pressure therapy in Asian obstructive sleep apnea. J Clin Sleep Med 2021;17(1):23–9.

80. Turino C, de Batlle J, Woehrle H, et al. Management of continuous positive airway pressure treatment compliance using telemonitoring in obstructive sleep apnoea. Eur Respir J 2017;49(2):1601128.

81. Prigent A, Gentina T, Launois S, et al. [Telemonitoring in continuous positive airway pressure-treated patients with obstructive sleep apnoea syndrome: an algorithm proposal]. Rev Mal Respir 2020; 37(7):550–60.

82. Isetta V, Thiebaut G, Navajas D, et al. E-telemed 2013: Proceedings Fifth International Conference on E-Health, Telemedicine and Social Medicine 2013; 156-161. Nice, February 24 - March 1, 2013.

83. Lankford DA. Wireless CPAP patient monitoring: accuracy study. Telemed J E Health 2004;10(2):162–9.

84. DeMolles DA, Sparrow D, Gottlieb DJ, et al. A pilot trial of a telecommunications system in sleep apnea management. Med Care 2004;42:764–9.

85. Kwiatkowska M, Idzikowski A, Matthews L. Telehealth-based framework for supporting the treatment of obstructive sleep apnea. Stud Health Technol Inform 2009;143:478–83.

86. Fraysse JL, Delavillemarque N, Gasparutto B, et al. Home telemonitoring of CPAP: a feasibility study. Rev Mal Respir 2012;29:60–3.

87. Tung P, Levitzky YS, Wang R, et al. Obstructive and central sleep apnea and the risk of incident atrial fibrillation in a community cohort of men and women. J Am Heart Assoc 2017;6:e004500.

88. Jiang WP, Wang L, Lin Song Y. Titration and follow-up for home noninvasive positive pressure ventilation in chronic obstructive pulmonary disease: the potential role of Tele-monitoring and the Internet of things. Clin Respir J 2021. [Epub ahead of print].

89. Stepnowsky C, Zamora T, Barker R, et al. Accuracy of positive airway pressure device-measured apneas and hypopneas: role in treatment followup. Sleep Disord 2013;2013:314589.

90. Rotty MC, Mallet JP, Suehs CM, et al. Is the 2013 American Thoracic Society CPAP-tracking system algorithm useful for managing non-adherence in long-term CPAP-treated patients? Respir Res 2019;20(1):209.

91. Huang HC, Hillman DR, McArdle N. Control of OSA during automatic positive airway pressure titration in a clinical case series: predictors and accuracy of device download data. Sleep 2012; 35(9):1277.

92. Reiter J, Zleik B, Bazalakova M, et al. Residual events during use of CPAP: prevalence, predictors, and detection accuracy. J Clin Sleep Med 2016;12(8):1153–8.

93. Hwang D. Monitoring progress and adherence with positive airway pressure therapy for obstructive sleep apnea: the roles of telemedicine and mobile health applications. Sleep Med Clin 2016;11: 161–71.

94. Schwab RJ, Badr SM, Epstein LJ, et al. An official American Thoracic Society Statement: continuous positive airway pressure adherence tracking systems. The optimal monitoring strategies and outcome measures in adults. Am J Respir Crit Care Med 2013;188(5):613–20.

95. Singh J, Badr S, Epstein L, et al. Sleep telemedicine implementation guide. Darien, US: AASM; 2017.

96. Aardoom JJ, Loheide-Niesmann L, Ossebaard HC, et al. Effectiveness of eHealth interventions in improving treatment adherence for adults with obstructive sleep apnea: meta-analytic review. J Med Internet Res 2020;22(2):e16972.

97. Chen C, Wang J, Pang L, et al. Telemonitor care helps CPAP compliance in patients with obstructive sleep apnea: a systemic review and meta-analysis of randomized controlled trials. Ther Adv Chronic Dis 2020;11. 2040622320901625.

98. Anttalainen U, Melkko S, Hakko S, et al. Telemonitoring of CPAP therapy may save nursing time. Sleep Breath 2016;20:1–7.

99. Hostler JM, Sheikh KL, Andrada TF, et al. A mobile, web-based system can improve positive airway pressure adherence. J Sleep Res 2017;26(2):139–46.

100. Kotzian ST, Saletu MT, Schwarzinger A, et al. Pro-active telemedicine monitoring of sleep apnea treatment improves adherence in people with stroke- a randomized controlled trial (HOPES study). Sleep Med 2019;64:48–55.

101. Nilius G, Schroeder M, Domanski U, et al. Telemedicine improves continuous positive airway pressure adherence in stroke patients with obstructive sleep apnea in a randomized trial. Respiration 2019; 98(5):410–20.

102. Pépin JL, Jullian-Desayes I, Sapène M, et al. Multimodal remote monitoring of high cardiovascular risk patients with OSA initiating CPAP: a randomized trial. Chest 2019;155(4):730–9.

103. Fernandes M, Antunes C, Martinho C, et al. Evaluation of telemonitoring of continuous positive airway pressure therapy in obstructive sleep apnoea syndrome: TELEPAP pilot study. J Telemed Telecare 2019. 1357633X19875850.

104. Tamisier R, Treptow E, Joyeux-Faure M, et al. Impact of a multimodal telemonitoring intervention on CPAP adherence in symptomatic OSA and low cardiovascular risk: a randomized controlled trial. Chest 2020;158(5):2136–45.

105. Murase K, Tanizawa K, Minami T, et al. A randomized controlled trial of telemedicine for long-term sleep apnea continuous positive airway pressure management. Ann Am Thorac Soc 2020;17(3):329–37.

106. Bixler EO, Vgontzas AN, Ten Have T, et al. Effects of age on sleep apnea in men: I. Prevalence and severity. Am J Respir Crit Care Med 1998;157(1):144–8.

107. Newman AB, Foster G, Givelber R, et al. Progression and regression of sleep-disordered breathing with changes in weight: the Sleep Heart Health Study. Arch Intern Med 2005;165(20):2408–13.

108. Baig MM, Antonescu-Turcu A, Ratarasarn K. Impact of sleep telemedicine protocol in management of sleep apnea: a 5-year VA experience. Telemed J E Health 2016;22(5):458–62.

109. Murphie P, Paton R, Scholefield C, et al. Telesleep medicine review—patient and clinician experience. Eur Respir J 2014;44(58):P3283.

110. Dieltjens M, Braem M, Vroegop A, et al. Objectively measured vs. self-reported compliance during oral appliance therapy for sleep-disordered breathing. Chest 2013;144(5):1495–502.

111. Seibert PS, Valerio J, DeHaas CA. The concomitant relationship shared by sleep disturbances and type 2 diabetes: developing telemedicine as a viable treatment option. J Diabet Sci Technol 2013;7(6):1607–15.

112. Gellis ZD, Kenaley B, McGinty J, et al. Outcomes of a telehealth intervention for homebound older adults with heart or chronic respiratory failure: a randomized controlled trial. Gerontologist 2012;52(4):541–52.

113. Paré G, Jaana M, Sicotte C. Systematic review of home telemonitoring for chronic diseases: the evidence base. J Am Med Inform Assoc 2007;14:269–77.

114. Kelly JM, Schwamm LH, Bianchi MT. Sleep telemedicine: a survey study of patient preferences. ISRN Neurol 2012;2012:135329.

115. Stepnowsky CJ Jr, Marler MR, Ancoli-Israel S. Determinants of nasal CPAP compliance. Sleep Med 2002;3(3):239–47.

116. Stepnowsky CJ, Marler MR, Palau J, et al. Social-cognitive correlates of CPAP adherence in experienced users. Sleep Med 2006;7(4):350–6.

117. Ayas NT, Patel SR, Malhotra A, et al. Auto-titrating versus standard continuous positive airway pressure for the treatment of obstructive sleep apnea: results of a meta-analysis. Sleep 2004;27(2):249–53.

118. Bakker JP, Weaver TE, Parthasarathy S, et al. Adherence to CPAP: what should we be aiming for, and how can we get there? Chest 2019; 155(6):1272–87.

119. Bogan RK, Wells C. A randomized crossover trial of a pressure relief technology (SensAwake) in continuous positive airway pressure to treat obstructive sleep apnea. Sleep Disord 2017;2017:3978073.

120. Leseux L, Rossin N, Sedkaoui K, et al. Education of patients with sleep apnea syndrome: feasibility of a phone coaching procedure. Phone coaching and SAS. Rev Mal Respir 2012;29(1):40–6.

121. Sedkaoui K, Leseux L, Pontier S, et al. Efficiency of a phone coaching program on adherence to continuous positive airway pressure in sleep apnea hypopnea syndrome: a randomized trial. BMC Pulm Med 2015;15:102.

122. Kuna ST, Shuttleworth D, Chi L, et al. Web-based access to positive airway pressure usage with or without an initial financial incentive improves treatment use in patients with obstructive sleep apnea. Sleep 2015;38(8):1229–36.

123. Suarez-Giron M, Bonsignore MR, Montserrat JM. New organisation for follow-up and assessment of treatment efficacy in sleep apnoea. Eur Respir Rev 2019;28(153):190059.

124. Aloia MS, Smith K, Arnedt JT, et al. Brief behavioral therapies reduce early positive airway pressure discontinuation rates in sleep apnea syndrome: preliminary findings. Behav Sleep Med 2007;5: 89–104.

125. Aloia MS, Arnedt JT, Strand M, et al. Motivational enhancement to improve adherence to positive airway pressure in patients with obstructive sleep apnea: a randomized controlled trial. Sleep 2013; 36:1655–62.

126. Bandura A. Self-efficacy: toward a unifying theory of behavioral change. Psychol Rev 1977;84(2): 191–215.

127. Bourbeau J, Nault D, Dang-Tan T. Self-manage-ment and behaviour modification in COPD. Patient Educ Couns 2004;52(3):271–7.

128. Pittard J, Yarascavitch J, Jasko J, et al. The use of SleepMapper (a patient self-management applica-tion) improves CPAP adherence in Australian pa-tients. Koninklijke Philips N.V.; 2015. Available on request from Philips Respironics, Philadelphia.

129. Woehrle H, Arzt M, Graml A, et al. Effect of a pa-tient engagement tool on positive airway pres-sure adherence: analysis of a German healthcare provider database. Sleep Med 2018; 41:20–6.

130. Malhotra A, Crocker ME, Willes L, et al. Patient engagement using new technology to improve adherence to positive airway pressure therapy: a retrospective analysis. Chest 2018;153(4):843–50.

131. Engleman H, Stitt C, Creswick L, et al. Effects on CPAP use of a patient support mobile app. Eur Re-spir J 2018;52(Suppl 62):PA2257.

132. Woehrle H, Ficker JH, Graml A, et al. Telemedicine-based proactive patient management during posi-tive airway pressure therapy: impact on therapy termination rate. Somnologie (Berl) 2017;21(2): 121–7.

133. Hibbard JH, Stockard J, Mahoney ER, et al. Devel-opment of the Patient Activation Measure (PAM): conceptualizing and measuring activation in pa-tients and consumers. Health Serv Res 2004;39: 1005–26.

134. Drager LF, Malhotra A, Yan Y, et al, medXcloud Group. Adherence with positive airway pressure therapy for obstructive sleep apnea in developing vs. developed countries: a big data study. J Clin Sleep Med 2021;17(4):703–9.

135. Billiard A, Rohmer V, Roques M, et al. Telematic trans-mission of computerized blood glucose profiles for IDDM patients. Diabetes Care 1991;14:130–4.

136. Friedman RH, Kazis LE, Jette A, et al. A telecommunications system for monitoring and counseling patients with hypertension: impact on medication adherence and blood pressure control. Am J Hypertens 1996;9:285–92.

137. Schwamm LH, Audebert HJ, Amarenco P. Stroke recommendations for the implementation of tele-medicine within stroke systems of care: a policy statement from the American Heart Association. Stroke 2009;40:2635–60.

138. Gustafson DH, Hawkins R, Boberg E, et al. Impact of a patientcentered, computer-based health informa-tion/support system. Am J Prev Med 1999;16:1–9.

139. Appel LJ, Clark JM. Comparative effectiveness of weight-loss interventions in clinical practice. N Engl J Med 2011;365(21):1959–68.

140. Wang G, Zhang Z, Feng Y, et al. Telemedicine in the management of Type 2 diabetes mellitus. Am J Med Sci 2017;353(1):1–5.

141. Bashi N, Karunanithi M, Fatehi F, et al. Remote monitoring of patients with heart failure: an over-view of systematic reviews. J Med Internet Res 2017;19(1):e18.

142. Gregersen TL, Green A, Frausing E, et al. Do tele-medical interventions improve quality of life in pa-tients with COPD? A systematic review. Int J Chron Obstruct Pulmon Dis 2016;11:809–22.

143. Takahasi PY, Pecina JL, Upatising B, et al. A randomized controlled trial of telemonitoring in older adults with multiple health issues to prevent hospitalizations and emergency department visits. Arch Intern Med 2012;172(10):773–9.

144. Farré R, Navajas D, Montserrat JM. Is telemedicine a key tool for improving continuous positive airway pressure adherence in patients with sleep apnea? Am J Respir Crit Care Med 2018;197(1):12–4.

145. Sutherland K, Kairaitis K, Yee BJ, et al. From CPAP to tailored therapy for obstructive sleep apnoea. Multidiscip Respir Med 2018;13:44.

146. Ritterband LM, Thorndike FP, Gonder-Frederick LA, et al. Efficacy of an Internet-based behavioral inter-vention for adults with insomnia. Arch Gen Psychi-atry 2009;66(7):692–8.

147. Espie CA, Kyle SD, Williams C, et al. A randomized, placebocontrolled trial of online cognitive behav-ioral therapy for chronic insomnia disorder deliv-ered via an automated media-rich Web application. Sleep 2012;35(6):769–81.

148. Zia S, Fields BG. Sleep telemedicine: an emerging field's latest frontier. Chest 2016;149(6):1556–65.

149. Richards D, Bartlett DJ, Wong K, et al. Increased adherence to CPAP with a group cognitive behav-ioral treatment intervention: a randomized trial. Sleep 2007;30(5):635–40.

150. Stepnowsky C, Sarmiento KF, Amdur A. Weaving the internet of sleep: the future of patient-centric collaborative sleep health management using web-based platforms. Sleep 2015;38(8):1157–8.

151. Bros JS, Poulet C, Arnol N, et al. Acceptance of tel-emonitoring among patients with obstructive sleep apnea syndrome: how is the perceived interest by and for patients? Telemed J E Health 2018;24: 351–9.

152. Luz PLD. Telemedicine and the doctor/patient rela-tionship. Arq Bras Cardiol 2019;113:100–2.

153. Bruyneel M. Technical developments and clinical use of telemedicine in sleep medicine. J Clin Med 2016;5:116.

154. Russo JE, McCool RR, Davies LVA. Telemedicine: an analysis of cost and time savings. Telemed J E Health 2016;22(3):209–15.

155. Huang W, Lee P, Liu Y, et al. 0495 Prediction of obstructive sleep apnea using machine learning technique. Sleep 2018;41(S1):A186.

156. Huang WC, Lee P-L, Liu Y, et al. Support vector machine prediction of obstructive sleep apnea in

a large-scale Chinese clinical sample. Sleep 2020; 43(7):zsz295.

157. Freedman N. Doing it better for less: incorporating OSA management into alternative payment models. Chest 2019;155(1):227–33.

158. He K, Palen BN, Mattox EA, et al. Veteran preferences regarding wireless management of positive airway pressure for obstructive sleep apnea at a tertiary health-care system. Respir Care 2017; 62(3):357–62.

159. Mendelson M, Vivodtzev I, Tamisier R, et al. CPAP treatment supported by telemedicine does not improve blood pressure in high cardiovascular risk OSA patients: a randomized, controlled trial. Sleep 2014;37:1863–70.

160. McManus RJ, Mant J, Franssen M, et al. Efficacy of self-monitored blood pressure, with or without tele-monitoring, for titration of antihypertensive medication (TASMINH4): an unmasked randomised controlled trial. Lancet 2018;391(10124):949–59.

161. Dieltjens M, Vanderveken OM. Oral appliances in obstructive sleep apnea. Healthcare (Basel) 2019;7(4):E141.

162. Inspire sleep apnea innovation: table of contents. Available at: https://professionals.inspiresleep. com/bibliography/. Accessed April 5, 2021.

163. Mukherjee S, Patel SR, Kales SN, et al. An official American Thoracic Society statement: the importance of healthy sleep. Recommendations and future priorities. Am J Respir Crit Care Med 2015; 191:1450–8.

164. Khosla S, Deak MC, Gault D, et al. Consumer sleep technology: an American Academy of Sleep Medicine position statement. J Clin Sleep Med 2018; 14(5):877–80.

165. O'Donnell C, Ryan S, McNicholas WT. The Impact of telehealth on the organization of the health system and integrated care. Sleep Med Clin 2020; 15(3):431–40.

166. Isetta V, Torres M, González K, et al. A New mHealth application to support treatment of sleep apnoea patients. J Telemed Telecare 2017;23(1): 14–8.

167. Ko PR, Kientz JA, Choe EK, et al. Consumer sleep technologies: a review of the landscape. J Clin Sleep Med 2015;11(12):1455–61.

168. Peleg M, Michalowski W, Wilk S, et al. Ideating mobile health behavioral support for compliance to therapy for patients with chronic disease: a case study of atrial fibrillation management. J Med Syst 2018;42(11):234.

169. Schiza S, Simonds A, Randerath W. Sleep laboratories reopening and COVID-19: a European perspective. Eur Respir J 2020;57(3):2002722.

170. Grote L, McNicholas WT, Hedner J, et al. Sleep apnoea management in Europe during the COVID-19 pandemic: data from the European sleep apnoea database (ESADA). Eur Respir J 2020;55(6):2001323.

171. Bonsignore MR, Baiamonte P, Mazzuca E, et al. Obstructive sleep apnea and comorbidities: a dangerous liaison. Multidiscip Respir Med 2019; 14:8.

172. Irfan M, Khalil W, Iber C. Practicing sleep medicine amidst a pandemic: a paradigm shift. J Clin Sleep Med 2020;16(8):1405–8.

173. Verbraecken J. Telemedicine applications in sleep disordered breathing: thinking out of the box. Sleep Med Clin 2016;11(4):445–59.

The Future of Sleep Measurements
A Review and Perspective

Erna Sif Arnardottir, PhD[a,b,]*, Anna Sigridur Islind, PhD[a,c],
María Óskarsdóttir, PhD[a,c]

KEYWORDS

- Sleep measurement • Subjective data • Objective data • Sleep diary • Codesign
- Machine learning • Data management platform • Data science

KEY POINTS

- This article argues for the need for improved subjective and objective assessment for future sleep studies and discusses the current use, limitations, and potentials of various types of sleep assessment.
- Data from wearables and nonwearables outline a future potential for informing sleep research and clinical practice to assess long-term effects on sleep, but these devices need to be validated further.
- Codesigning with patients and health care professionals can enable improved diagnostics and collaborative care, informed by data.
- Data management platforms designed and developed to securely display a variety of data for (1) health care professionals, (2) patients, and (3) researchers can enable the synergy of objective and subjective data in 1 place.
- Data science and machine learning techniques applied to a variety of sleep data can facilitate the discovery of new and important patterns and novel insights in sleep data.

INTRODUCTION

Sleep assessment depends both on the subjective experience of the individual and objective measurements, which are traditionally collected through an overnight sleep study. In addition, wearable and nonwearable devices are increasingly being used to collect objective data over a longer period and thus offer new ways to assess sleep and its long-term effect on health and well-being. The various types of data all tell an important story for the sleep diagnosis because each type represents a different side of the same coin. Therefore, to have the most complete picture of someone's sleep, these various types of data need to be considered and analyzed, as has been shown in other areas of research as well.[1]

DIFFERENT TECHNIQUES TO MEASURE SLEEP
Subjective Assessment

A crucial part of a sleep assessment is the subjective experience of the patient, which in many cases is sufficient to make a clinical diagnosis without the need for any objective sleep testing. This stage includes the diagnosis and treatment of, for example, insomnia (difficulties initiating or maintaining sleep) and restless legs syndrome (an urge to move legs and/or uncomfortable/unpleasant[2] sensation in legs) as well as numerous other sleep disorders.[3] For other disorders, such as obstructive sleep apnea (OSA), the subjective experience of the patient is usually very limited. People typically only knows that they snore or have apneas during sleep if told by a bed partner.

[a] Reykjavik University Sleep Institute, School of Technology, Reykjavik University, Menntavegi 1, 102 Reykjavik, Iceland; [b] Internal Medicine Services, Landspitali University Hospital, E7 Fossvogi, 108 Reykjavik, Iceland;
[c] Department of Computer Science, Reykjavik University, Menntavegi 1, 102 Reykjavik, Iceland
* Corresponding author. Reykjavik University, Menntavegi 1, 102 Reykjavik, Iceland.
E-mail address: ernasifa@ru.is

Sleep Med Clin 16 (2021) 447–464
https://doi.org/10.1016/j.jsmc.2021.05.004
1556-407X/21/© 2021 Elsevier Inc. All rights reserved.

Therefore, in OSA, an objective sleep measurement is necessary for diagnosis.[3] The subjective part is often overlooked and dismissed as less important than objective measurements of sleep, especially by those less experienced in the relevant sleep disorder.

Questionnaires

A vast number of questionnaires have been created in the last decades to assess sleep, sleep problems, and their effects on daytime functioning. Shahid and colleagues[4] reviewed more than 100 sleep questionnaires, and an extensive number of others are additionally used. At present, the most validated and popular screening questionnaire for OSA is the STOP-Bang, which stands for Snoring, Tiredness, Observed apnea, blood Pressure, Body mass index, Age, Neck circumference and Gender.[5–8] The list of available OSA screening questionnaires is much larger and includes the Berlin questionnaire[9] and The Neck, Obesity, Snoring, Age, Sex (NoSAS) questionnaire.[10] Le Grande and colleagues[11] identified 21 instruments designed to assess the likelihood of OSA in cardiac patients. To assess excessive daytime sleepiness, the Epworth Sleepiness Scale[12–14] is the most popular, but others, such as the Karolinska Sleepiness Scale[15] and Stanford Sleepiness Scale,[16] are also widely used. For overall sleep quality, the Pittsburgh Sleep Quality Index,[17] with 19 items in 7 subcategories, is frequently used, but other exist as well.

Limitations Most sleep questionnaires are markedly flawed. Many of them are not properly validated against a diagnosis of a clinical sleep disorder, the asked time frame varies widely, and many use imprecise wording such as "Recently" and "Frequently" instead of using a specific time frame for answering. Also, often a "Don't know" option is not included.[18] This makes it difficult for many people to answer questions about occurrences during sleep such as snoring frequency and loudness, leg kicks, and other movements, especially for those who do not have a bed partner. It is then impossible to know whether a person forgot to answer or did not know how to answer specific questions. Other questions may be poorly designed because they ask about more than 1 issue in the same questions. For example, in the Pittsburgh Sleep Quality Index, the question "During the past month, how often have you had trouble sleeping because you cough or snore loudly?" addresses 2 separate issues.

Some questionnaires are biased toward male responses. The Epworth Sleepiness Scale measures the ability to fall asleep or doze in different situations. The Epworth captures sleepiness better for men, relating more strongly with reported feelings of sleepiness or being unrested, than for women.[19] Women also less often have a total Epworth score greater than 10, which is the clinical cutoff for excessive daytime sleepiness, despite women reporting feeling sleepy as often as men.[19] Women are less likely to report classic OSA symptoms such as snoring and witnessed apneas than men.[20] However, they are more likely than men to report tiredness, sleep onset insomnia, and morning headaches.[20] The results of this are numerous, including screening questionnaires such as the STOP-Bang being less sensitive to female OSA and the need for sex-specific screening.[21] STOP-Bang additionally has 1 extremely poorly worded question: "Gender = Male? Yes or No." In the authors experience, many women are offended by the setup of this question and a better-worded question for addressing gender in modern society is needed.[22]

In addition, the reliability and validity of different sleep questionnaires have often been assessed to a limited extent.[4,23] Reliability assessment includes internal consistency, test-retest reliability, and, when appropriate, interrater reliability. The validity assessment includes content and construct validity. A questionnaire that has been validated, for example, in a general population may have very different sensitivity and specificity to detect the relevant sleep problem than in a sleep clinic population.[23] The format of the questionnaire is important as well, whether it is administered by interview or is self-administered using paper-and-pencil or digital format.[4,24]

To capture the different aspects needed to understand a person's sleep pattern, a clinician or researcher needs to mix and match from the large number of available questionnaires.[4] For example, several different questionnaires are needed to assess a person's regular sleep-wake patterns and daytime sleepiness, as well as to screen for common sleep disorders such as OSA and insomnia. Other important items, such a smoking history, exercise level, caffeine consumption, comorbidities, and medication, need to be assessed by a different set of questions. Therefore, the patient burden is increased with longer times to answer repetitive questions in different sections and with varying question formats and instructions in a single test battery. Some efforts to develop a common test battery based on compilation of questionnaires, such as the Sleep Apnea Global Interdisciplinary Consortium questionnaire[25] and the Western Australian Sleep Health Study Questionnaire, have been published, but validation of their psychometric properties is still lacking.

Future potential Most questionnaires are currently designed for paper-and-pencil answering, and intermethod reliability needs to be validated for digital format. Also, designing questionnaires specifically for digital format allows a different structure for follow-up questions. For example, now a broad general question about a specific category can be asked. If the patient has no perceived issues in the category, the patient can move on to the next category, but if an issue is detected, a much deeper probing can be performed. Also, further screening questionnaire development such as the STOP-Bang and NoSAS score,[10] designed to exclude OSA in patients who have low probability of disease and do not need further objective testing, is needed. The reliability and validity of further questionnaire development need to be assessed for different populations, including clinical and general population, women and men separately, as well as in different ethnic groups and age categories. These questionnaires should be codesigned with both patients and health care workers (details are discussed later) and be reviewed thoroughly by relevant experts for the different design flaws described earlier.

Interviews

The gold-standard sleep assessment includes an interview with a qualified sleep physician (or somnologist). European standards indicate a 1-hour interview with a sleep physician to review patient history, a physical examination, and review of questionnaires.[26] The importance of conducting a detailed clinical interview including a physical examination is highlighted in the *Sleep Medicine Textbook* of the European Sleep Research Society (ESRS).[27] The American Academy of Sleep Medicine (AASM) has also provided a detailed list of screening questions for the sleep history and physical examination on their Web site. However, who is responsible for this text, the date of publication, and whether the interview has been validated are unclear.[28] The structure and length of the clinical interview are likely to differ widely between countries and sleep laboratories.

A few structured interviews, including the Diagnostic Interview for Sleep Patterns and Disorders (DISP),[29] the Structured Clinical Interview for Sleep Disorders (SCISD), and the Diagnostic and Statistical Manual of Mental Disorders, Fifth Edition (DSM-5),[30] have been generated. These interviews can be administered by a trained interviewer without sleep expertise, take about 10 to 30 minutes, and have been validated to some extent.[29,30]

Limitations Access to a qualified sleep physician is scarce and waiting lists worldwide for clinical interviews are typically very long. Therefore, most patients with sleep problems will never meet such a specialist. Further validation of structured interviews that can be administered by trained non–sleep experts is needed to facilitate a wider use of such instruments.

Future potential The generation of a simple-to-use, clinically validated structured clinical interview as a test battery for a variety of sleep problems to improve patient care is greatly needed. This clinical interview needs to assess sleep hygiene, insomnia, delayed sleep phase, OSA as well as other potential sleep disorders. Such a tool would allow general practitioners, cardiologists, psychologists, and other health care professionals to thoroughly assess a person's sleep profile and direct patients to the needed diagnostics tests and treatments to improve their sleep. Patients with continued problems could then be referred to a more specialized sleep expert. The structured clinical interview would preferably be available online, free of charge, for all health care professionals to use, providing automatic calculations of the risk for different sleep disorders, with guidelines for health care professionals for the next steps. In addition, a comparison between the validity of a structured clinical interview and a digital self-administered questionnaire with the same items would be advisable. If a digital questionnaire has similar validity to the structured clinical interview, valuable health care personnel time can then be saved for other purposes.

The authors would also like to emphasize the need for in-depth, structured, or semistructured interviews, observations, and focus groups to gather empirical data to improve the different tools used for subjective measurements described in this article. These interviews and focus groups transcripts could then be analyzed through thematic analysis, or through content analysis,[31] to shed light on new patterns in sleep disorders or subjective feelings that could be revealed through such data gathering. Thematic analysis includes closely examining the data to identify recurrent and common themes. These themes can consist of topics, ideas, or patterns that arise frequently. Although the process can differ, typically it is divided into 6 phases: (1) familiarization, (2) coding, (3) generating themes, (4) reviewing themes, (5) defining and naming themes, and (6) writing up.[31–33]

Sleep diaries

Sleep diaries have an important role in the diagnosis and treatment monitoring of insomnia and another sleep disorders, such as circadian rhythm disturbances.[34] The typical sleep diary is used for 1 to 2 weeks to assess a person's overall sleep length, timing, and quality, as well as factors that may affect sleep, such as daytime naps, sleeping pills, and caffeine and alcohol use. The persons answering then estimate the previous night's sleep the following morning by answering questions about when they went to bed, how long it took them to fall asleep and whether they woke up during the night. The sleep diary gives an important overview to the sleep expert of the overall subjective sleep experience of the patient or research subject.

However, there is also a consensus regarding the need to standardize sleep diaries, because many different versions are available and used by different sleep experts.[35,36] There are various aspects that vary currently within the literature reporting on sleep diaries: (1) the wording of questions, (2) the number of questions, (3) the format of delivery (**Fig. 1**), (4) the duration of the data collection (typically performed for 1–2 weeks but can vary), (5) answering once or twice per day, and (6) whether it should be paper-and-pencil or digital format.[36–38] Therefore, the generation of the Consensus Sleep Diary in 2012[36] was a major step toward standardization of this important tool.

Limitations Even the Consensus Sleep Diary generated by an expert panel includes 3 different versions, with a core part designed to fit 2 sides of a single sheet of paper and an extended, optional version.[36] Focus group feedback indicated that some participants preferred a graphical format, such as clock faces or time charts. Also, participants commented that specific aspects of the sleep of a given night could not be well described.[36] Therefore, as indicated by the investigators, further ways to standardize and improve sleep diary assessment are needed.

An important limitation to sleep diaries is compliance; that is, the participants may forget to fill in the sleep diary. Some patients and research participants may then attempt to fill in entries for several days in a row, which is especially bad in a paper-and-pencil format where there is no way to know when the participant did the assessment. Another limitation is the subjective nature of the sleep diary, which can be affected by, for example, memory bias.

Future potential Future possibilities could include sleep diaries in mobile applications (or apps). Using smartphones to deliver sleep diaries through mobile apps could be a way to (1) ensure more compliance in answering through nudging the participants with screen notifications, (2) know when the participants fill in the sleep diaries, and (3) limiting when an event can be registered. An additional aspect that could be added to sleep diaries is the impact of continuous self-assessment on patient self-care and empowerment, by evaluating whether the participants change their lifestyles over time, through being asked about their lifestyles every day. Future possibilities include adding questions about the subjective experience of the participants

Name of patient: Andrea	Date: 26/03/2021
1. What time did you get into bed?	22:35
2. What time did you try to go to sleep	23:00
3. How long did it take you to fall asleep?	15 min.
4. How many times did you wake up, not counting your final awakening?	2 times
5. In total, how long did these awakenings last?	40 min.
6. What time was your final awakening?	07:00
7. What time did you get out of bed for the day?	07:15

Fig. 1. Examples of 2 different types of sleep diary, 1 with a quantitative approach where the patient needs to fill in specific times in hours and minutes, and a qualitative approach where the patient fills in approximate times in a visual sleep diary.

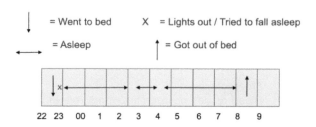

and regular objective alertness tests. This addition could give patients insight into how different aspects, such as short sleep duration, affect their next-day functioning or how excessive caffeine/alcohol use affects their next night's sleep.

Objective Assessment

The number of objective ways to assess sleep and sleep disorders is high (**Fig. 2**). The gold-standard diagnostic method is generally considered to be an in-laboratory polysomnogram (PSG).[39,40] However, this method is not the right tool for every sleep problem and cannot measure the subjective experiences of the patients, as described earlier. A PSG without any subjective information in many cases does not yield any meaningful clinical results; for example, for the diagnosis of insomnia.[3]

Type 1 to 4 sleep studies

The gold-standard sleep study is considered an attended, in-laboratory PSG, or type 1 sleep study.[2] This study refers to the patient sleeping

in a hospital or laboratory environment, monitored by staff the whole night to ensure the quality of the study. The study includes 6 channels to measure electroencephalography (EEG) for brain wave activity, left and right electrooculography (EOG) to measure eye movements, and chin electromyography (EMG) for muscle tone. Two reference channels are added on the mastoid bone behind both ears for the EEG and EOG assessments. Together, the EEG, EOG, and EMG allow the assessment of different sleep stages and wake periods measured in 30-second epochs throughout the night and arousals from sleep. PSG also includes respiratory flow assessment via a nasal cannula and thermistor to assess nasal and mouth breathing. Respiratory movements are measured via thorax and abdomen belts and oxygen saturation via pulse oximeter. Together, these measurements allow the assessment of sleep apnea severity and subtypes (obstructive, mixed, or central). In addition, an electrocardiography (ECG) test, leg EMG (for periodic leg movement assessment), body

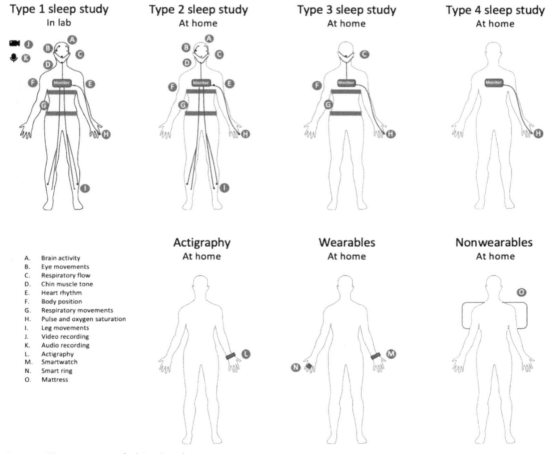

A. Brain activity
B. Eye movements
C. Respiratory flow
D. Chin muscle tone
E. Heart rhythm
F. Body position
G. Respiratory movements
H. Pulse and oxygen saturation
I. Leg movements
J. Video recording
K. Audio recording
L. Actigraphy
M. Smartwatch
N. Smart ring
O. Mattress

Fig. 2. Different types of objective sleep measurements.

position, and synchronized video and audio are included. The PSG is manually edited or scored for different events, including sleep stages, arousals, respiratory events, and periodic leg movements. This scoring is described in detail in *The AASM Manual for the Scoring of Sleep and Associated Events*,[39] the most widely used standard for sleep scoring, although some major differences exist in scoring standards worldwide that affect all attempts for automation of sleep scoring. For more details, see review articles.[41,42]

Other types of objective sleep studies are referred to as home sleep apnea testing by the AASM. Therefore, this term includes every type of sleep study performed at home/portable, which are very diverse. Another terminology that is more detailed is type 1 to type 4 sleep studies. Type 1 is an attended in-laboratory PSG and types 2 to 4 are described next and in **Fig. 2**.

A type 2 sleep study is a home PSG that includes all the same channels as an in-laboratory PSG except for the video recording, and, depending on the device used, an audio recording may or may not be included. Typically, the patient goes to the sleep laboratory, where a sleep technologist sets up the study (takes about 1 hour), and the patient is then sent home to sleep.[39]

A type 3 sleep study is also called a polygraphy, portable monitoring, or cardiorespiratory study. A type 3 study has the same channels as are recorded in a PSG, excluding the sensor required for sleep measurement (EEG, EOG, and chin EMG). The study comprises sensors to assess breathing, oxygen saturation, pulse, and body position. In some devices, additional sensors, such as ECG and leg EMG, can be added. Type 3 sleep studies are currently considered for OSA diagnostics in patients with a high pretest probability.[39] However, the definition of what is considered a high pretest probability is often not clearly stated.[40] Some articles have defined a high pretest probability using OSA screening questionnaires, which have marked flaws, as discussed earlier.[43,44]

A type 4 sleep study involves limited-channel monitoring with 1 to 3 parameters. One type 4 study, which includes peripheral arterial tone (PAT), pulse oximetry, and wrist activity, is accepted by the AASM.[39] Guidelines from the ESRS and Assembly of the National Sleep Societies (ANSS) in Europe do not accept the use of such studies for a final diagnosis of any sleep disorders, although an update of these guidelines is needed because they are now almost 10 year old.[26]

Limitations A major limitation to all sleep studies is that they are typically only applied for a single night, both for clinical and research studies. Therefore night-to-night variability in different sleep parameters and the potential first-night effect of sleeping with a device are not measured.[45–47] Type 1 studies have also been criticized as the gold-standard measurement because of the unnatural sleep environment of the patients, who are expected to sleep normally during 1 night in a hospital environment with none of the normal home routines for the evening or night. Also, because of the number of wires attached to the patient and often to a device on the bedside, patients may sleep more in the supine position than normally. This position can, for example, increase OSA severity in patients with supine OSA to clinical levels, although the patients only sleep nonsupine at home.[48] Type 2 to 4 sleep studies are more likely to have some quality issues than type 1 studies, because some issues may come up before the patient goes to sleep and/or during the night and they are not continuously monitored.[49] Type 3 and 4 sleep studies lack measurement of sleep. Therefore, the total sleep time and wake periods cannot be assessed except in some devices via surrogate markers.[50,51] Also, phenotypes such as rapid eye movement–related OSA cannot be assessed.[46,47] Further work to convince most sleep clinicians that these surrogate markers are adequate to measure sleep on an epoch-by-epoch basis are needed.[42] Also, arousals as markers of sleep fragmentation cannot be assessed, which additionally affects the scoring of other events; for example, hypopneas followed by arousals without oxygen desaturation,[39] which affect the measured OSA severity. Type 4 sleep studies then additionally lack measurement of respiration and rely on surrogate markers to assess breathing stops and typically rely on automatic analysis, although some efforts for manual scoring have started.[50] Type 4 sleep studies relying on PAT technology have on average a very high accuracy compared with PSG,[52] but care should be taken with individual patient results, which can differ extensively from the gold-standard measurement. Again, event-by-event comparison needs to be performed and published to adequately validate this technology. Furthermore, special care needs to be taken with patients with different comorbidities and medication use in choosing relevant patients for both type 3 and type 4 sleep studies, again highlighting the role of a thorough subjective assessment.[2]

In addition, type 3 and type 4 studies can be marked by the so-called law of the instrument,[53] namely being over-reliant on a familiar tool or a narrow skill set, especially for physicians who are not sleep specialists and have a limited knowledge of other sleep disorders or how to screen for them. Performing such a sleep study may result in incidental findings of OSA, which are not the main symptom of the patient.[41]

Future potential Some efforts have been made to create self-applied PSGs,[54–56] which the patients can then apply themselves at home, saving valuable clinic time. Self-applied PSG could also allow continued sleep services during periods such as the coronavirus disease 2019 (COVID-19) epidemic, which mostly halted in-laboratory services and PSG setups.[57] However, self-applied setups do require extensive testing before their acceptance in clinical use. The EEG is typically located only on the forehead (F channels), with no electrodes located on the top of the scalp (C channels) and back of the head (O channels) as in traditional PSG.[39] Research on the number of failed sleep studies and a quality review of signals compared with home PSG set up by a sleep technologist needs to be done, as well as patient feedback collected for optimizing the setup (details are discussed later). Self-applied setups could also facilitate the use of multinight studies to capture night-to-night variability and would then be less costly than in-laboratory or home PSG set up by sleep technologists.

In an era when clinicians have started to rethink many of the current standards used in sleep scoring, such as the fixed 30-second sleep epoch[58] and the counting of respiratory events by the apnea-hypopnea index to measure OSA severity,[41,59] type 3 and type 4 studies may have limited value in the future because they were validated against potentially outdated diagnostic tests. A type 1 or 2 PSG is important for current research purposes to better understand the essential signals needed for improved future sleep diagnostics.

Actigraphy
To assess so-called free-living sleep conditions, multiple-night recordings in the home environment need to be performed.[60] Actigraphy studies outline a methodological approach for inferring both sleep and wake patterns primarily based on movement data from small sensors.[61] In the medical field, studies that use actigraphy are typically accomplished by using a wrist actigraph, a small watch-like device embedding an accelerometer and that often also records ambient light and skin temperature.[60] The use of actigraphy is accompanied by a subjective sleep diary such as those discussed earlier. Clinical guidelines recommend that the patient wears the actigraph for 7 to 14 days, but 72 hours of recording is generally sufficient to bill

for the testing in the United States.[60] For research purposes, 5 to 7 days of actigraphy measurement is also often used to assess sleeping behavior.[62] These data can then be used to assess, for example, average sleep duration, chronotype (morningness vs eveningness), and other sleep parameters of interest.

Limitations In an epoch-by-epoch validation study of actigraphy against PSG, it was shown that they are a useful and valid means for estimating total sleep time and wakefulness after sleep onset but are limited in terms of specificity.[63] Also, actigraphy does not measure sleep stages or arousals. In studies with actigraphy, patients need to always wear the watch, while also keeping a sleep diary, which requires high compliance.[64] False-positives are also common; that is, the watch is good at detecting sleep but worse at detecting wakefulness.[63] In addition, actigraphy is prone to technical malfunctions, which can entail lost data that will not be discovered until the patient or research participant returns the device for downloading.[64]

Future potential A systematic literature review showed that the accuracy of actigraphy devices is often not significantly different from PSG, but they have a high variability for the same individual. In contrast, EEG-based devices are both more accurate and have less variability, whereas devices that measure behavioral aspects of sleep onset consistently overestimated their PSG counterparts.[65] Because actigraphy essentially uses wearable devices, there is much potential in equipping them with additional functionalities, such as sweating and heart rate variability or even using them as an addition to other type of wearables. However, adding any additional measure could improve their accuracy but would require them to be validated again.

Wearables and nonwearables
Self-trackers collect vital signs, including sleep measurements, on a continuous basis for millions of individuals in an unprecedented way. Wearable technology is an umbrella term for body-worn sensors with the ability to send and receive data that can be exchanged between the sensor and a network, such as smartwatches, which capture the same information as an actigraphy while also collecting a wider range of physiologic signal data, such as pulse.[66–68] Other connected devices, called nonwearables, are placed in a location near the body and used to monitor physiologic signals (for example, connected mattresses to monitor sleep patterns).[69] These are increasingly used in conjunction with wearables

in health-related research studies.[70,71] The use of wearable and nonwearable self-trackers is becoming increasingly popular among the general public for personal monitoring of health and fitness and to measure vital signs on a continuous basis. As such, the devices are collecting unprecedented volumes of individuals' vital signs at a granular level, including movements, physical activity, step count, heart rate, sleep duration, and sleep quality, 24 hours a day, 7 days a week. The devices typically come with a mobile application, designed and distributed by the company that produces the self-trackers, where the users can see their various measurements and trends over time. In some cases, aggregated data can be retrieved for research purposes with the consent of the participants.

Limitations To assess the capabilities and accuracy of self-trackers to measure sleep, they need to be validated. To achieve this, they are compared with the gold-standard PSG or actigraphy in a double setup either in a clinical setting or free-living environment for 1 to 3 nights.[72–74] Numerous validation studies exist, as well as a few meta-studies that systematically investigate the results of such validation studies. The results show that wearables tend to overestimate sleep time and sleep efficiency compared with PSG.[75,76] A systematic review of wearables' estimation of sleep onset showed that the estimate is adequate.[77,78] Further epoch-by-epoch analysis of sleep stages and event-by-event analysis of, for example, breathing stops is needed to validate these devices and for them to be accepted in clinical use.

It is worth noting that these sensors, independent of whether they are body worn or kept close to the body, are consumer products that are designed and developed for the general public and not for specific sleep disorders or for treatment purposes. The same holds for the accompanying digital platforms. What is concerning is that there are no standards, neither regarding the way the data is collected nor in the way the data are analyzed and visualized, for the customers using the self-trackers. The algorithms used to analyze the data are black boxes that are usually not disclosed because they are considered business secrets in this competitive market.[65] There is a certain secrecy in the way the companies estimate sleep stages, and the sleep stage estimation varies between the companies, so, depending on the company's definition behind the algorithms, the sleep stage can vary. In addition, processes and algorithms are frequently updated without the knowledge of the user, which means that the results shown in the

digital platform may not be comparable over time. Moreover, there is an algorithmic bias[79] in the analysis generated by the companies providing the sensors. However, if each participant wears the same device through the entirety of a study, and as long as devices of the same type are compared, they can be useful.

Another point of importance is the potential for such self-trackers to induce anxiety or obsession with sleep with an overreliance on these data. This anxiety can cause the nicely coined orthosomnia.[80]

In addition, there is a clear discrepancy between the various types of self-trackers in the way they collect data and display it to the user.[81] What is also alarming is the gap between the sleep community and the wearable technology companies regarding the way sleep is measured and communicated to the user. This gap could be bridged with more communication between the stakeholders and adoption of standard metrics for validation of consumer self-trackers.[65]

Future potential Self-trackers collect vital signs, including sleep measurements, on a continuous basis for millions of individuals in an unprecedented way. Although the devices are designed for personal monitoring, people are sharing their measurements with their physicians. Given proper guidelines and standards in addition to insightful visualization and meaningful statistical summaries of the various measurements, they could interpret events and trends in the data and use them in decision support for the patients' care. Properly validated wearables and nonwearables will allow clinicians to assess changes in sleep patterns over extended periods, including seasonal effects on sleep[82] and sleep apnea severity.[83] Changes with age and weight increase, alcohol and caffeine intake, exercise, and so forth can then also be studied in much more detail than current measures allow. If this is done in conjunction with sleep diaries and questionnaires, valuable data on sleep can be collected from any given individual. When using wearables and nonwearables, the sensors generate low-resolution data.[84] Consequently, because the data from these sensors do not capture all the vital signs that a PSG does, the data gathering needs to include an extended period of time.

TOOLS FOR MAXIMIZING FUTURE SLEEP MEASUREMENTS
Data Management Platform

The term digital platform indicates that the platform is a piece of software relying on resilient hardware, although it is also an intermediary that connects needs with resources, sellers with customers, users with service providers, or patients with health care professionals.[85,86] A digital platform is an organizational, technical, and regulatory construct that facilitates value exchange and value creation. Such constructs are especially interesting in a health care context to facilitate data exchange and data sharing. The types of digital platforms, where the main objective is data sharing, are termed data management platforms.

For data management platforms to be used in sleep research, 4 main aspects are of importance. These aspects are scalability, layered-modular architecture, security, and level of access. Regarding scalability, the era of big data is pushing the limits of size. Big data is now not merely an impressive, exciting concept of the future; instead, that age has already arrived, gathering big data on patients and research participants for health care purposes.[87] To handle this scalability, the literature suggests designing and developing the infrastructure of data management platforms through a layered-modular architectural approach.[88,89] Such architecture entails dividing the platform into a content layer, service layer, network layer, and device layer. To date, digital platforms have mostly been designed, developed, and used for 2 main purposes: (1) development platforms, and (2) transaction platforms, and the architecture of them shares similar characteristics, such as the layers outlined earlier. Development platforms are designed for the purpose of facilitating app development, whereas transaction platforms are designed for the purpose of facilitating various types of transactions,[90] where 1 such transaction can be data. Less focus has been on the design and development of digital platforms meant for health care settings and designed for the purpose of sharing data specifically. However, the literature on digital platforms where the main transaction is data is growing.[86]

Limitations

In health care, a large area of improvement is needed in relation to security and level of access while sharing data in general and while sharing the various types of data, such as those specified in this article, which vary in size, granularity, and type. In addition to that, the data discussed herein originate from various types of sensors and devices, which makes the sharing of data, to a shared location, increasingly complex, and that is where security and level of access come in. In addition, sharing data between end-user groups with diverse needs is also a known limitation of most health care systems. For example, the electronic patient record is designed to serve a documenting and administrating purpose for health care professionals but has been further extended to include sharing options for patients accessing data, at least in some countries. This divergence in design versus use is not optimal. Instead, it is important to define the end users into stakeholder groups upfront and to structure the architectural choices accordingly. Few attempts have been successfully executed where data can be securely shared between researchers, health care professionals, and patients through the same digital platform within health care, where the level of access is controlled carefully, and that is where the potential of data management platforms comes in.

Future potential

Future potentials include designing and developing secure data management platforms for sharing data on sleep between 3 main types of end users: (1) researchers, (2) health care professionals, and (3) patients and research participants. These end-user groups then have access to a subset of the data, depending on their level of access. This type of architecture can be used to support research through connecting various kinds of data, collected by health care professionals and patients into 1 common place. That is why the authors argue that data management platforms are at the nexus of where the future of sleep research and sleep measurements will be, with secure layered-modular architecture and tight access control. Furthermore, data management platforms can be used to display a variety of data, gathered through different types of devices and methods, in the same platform. Also, the same data presentation for devices from different manufacturers can then be visualized to facilitate their easier use for health care professionals, focusing on the information needs of this end-user type.

Importance of Codesign and Cocare

There is a history of failed implementations of large-scale digital infrastructures in health care settings. These digital infrastructures have been pushed down the organizations in a top-down manner, and 1 such example is electronic patient records, which suffer from usability issues in most countries.[91–93] Based on that, when designing and developing digital technology, such as the data management platforms elaborated on earlier, with the purpose of supporting everyday life and work, the design processes can differ substantially. The design process can on the one hand be done with detachment from the end users (ie, the designated users of the digital technology), of which the electronic patient record is a famous example, or, in contrast, the design process can be conducted through engagement with the end users.[86]

There has been a long-standing focus on end-user participation and engagement in the design process in research,[94] whereas, in practice, the detachment paradigm is sometimes considered the most effective way forward in costly processes of large-scale digital innovation. However, the authors argue that, when designing and developing digital technology to support a group of heterogenous end users, the most effective way in coping with the complexity of the needs of the various stakeholder groups is through end-user engagement.[95] When involving the end users, there must be a dual focus on empowerment of the end users and on generating focused ideas that can be handed over to the developers. This process can be done through codesign.

Codesign refers to a collaborative creative activity where end users, who are not trained in design work, engage with designers on ideas in order to further the design process and thus incorporate the specific needs of the end users early on.[96] More specifically, in codesign, the design process is regarded as a specific aspect of cocreation where the end users are engaged as codesigners (ie, as collaborative agents or actors in the design process) where it is essential that the end users are seen as a valuable resource to further the design process.[96] Involving the end users in design is not new. In participatory design, it has been the guiding philosophy for half a decade. An important building block in the move toward participatory design was written in 1972.[97] The fundamentals of codesign as an approach thereby entail the end users having a voice in the design processes that ultimately affect their lives.[98,99] In health care settings, where patients, health care professionals, and researchers intersect and use the same digital infrastructure, in different ways, there is the need to involve representatives from each of those end-user groups, and not just 1.

When selecting end users as codesigners in the care for frail patients, context-related issues can be created, such as those related to identity. Accordingly, in a successful codesign process, where patients are involved, it is vital that the end users can identify themselves as the future end users of the digital technology that is being designed,[100,101] and that the selection of representatives (ie, codesigners) is diverse.[95] In addition, the codesign process can set the scene for cocare, where the patients are participants in their own care to a larger extent because the digital infrastructure was designed by them, for them.[85,95] Studies also show that health care professionals who regard the same system as their own, designed by and for them, are more likely to accept the system and the change it entails.[95]

Limitations

The main limitation of involving various types of stakeholders is time. It takes time to meet with the representatives of the end users repeatedly and show them new developments in the design, get their feedback, and iterate that feedback into the design. The iterations take time, time that pays off in the long run, but still slows down the process in the beginning.[99] Another known limitation is leveraging various needs and knowing when to favor, for example, the health care professionals rather than the patients, or vice versa, when they have conflicting views on the design.[95]

Future potentials

The way the design process is orchestrated and organized is essential to the outcome and acceptance of the digital infrastructure in the long run. Facilitating the collaboration between the patients and their health care professionals early on can function as a basis for understanding the future use situation and can foster acceptance for the system, and for the change. Conclusively, design approaches, such as codesign, where genuine user participation is key in the design process, also have to consider the frail end users and their specific needs in a codesign process, while catering to the needs of the health care professionals and ultimately researchers. This requirement makes the complexity high, but a change is needed, for example, in the development of subjective measurements of sleep, and the results will likely improve greatly the tools for both clinical and research needs, in a process such as shown in **Fig. 3**.

IMPROVED SLEEP DATA ANALYSIS

The different types of sleep data available, as described earlier, vary greatly; for example, in terms of subjective versus objective nature, granularity, frequency, timespan, amount of noise and data quality. To extract knowledge and insights from the data, there are several methods, processes, algorithms, and systems are classed under interdisciplinary data science, also known as data mining and analytics, including preprocessing the data by removing noise and errors, extracting and engineering useful and informative variables from structured and unstructured data, finding correlations between different measurements and events, summarizing main aspects of the data to give an overview, visualizing the data in insightful ways, and inspecting trends.[102] The

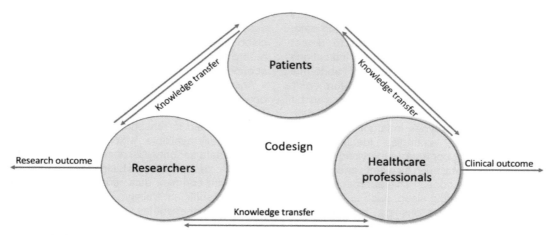

Fig. 3. Bedside-to-bench and bench-to-bedside: the power of knowledge transfer between researchers, health care professionals, and patients to improve both clinical and research outcomes.

cross-industry standard process model for data mining (CRISP-DM) is the most widely used model for these tasks and applies to any domain, including analysis of sleep data. It breaks the cyclic process into 6 phases that the practitioner is typically required to move back and forward between.[103] The process, shown in **Fig. 4**, usually begins with understanding the needs of the domain where the techniques will be deployed, together with an investigation of the available data. Once the relevant data have been selected, they must be prepared, which involves preprocessing and transforming them to obtain clean target data and having the relevant features extracted. Next comes the modeling phase, where

statistical and machine learning techniques are applied to discover insightful patterns. The resulting models are then evaluated to measure their performance and interpret the results. When the model is ready, it can be deployed and the insights that were gained from the process used to enhance the domain understanding.

A major component of data science is the modeling phase, which usually consists of machine learning; that is, algorithms that improve automatically through experience or by using large amounts of data to learn from. The main approaches in machine learning are unsupervised learning, supervised learning, and reinforcement learning.[102,104] Unsupervised learning is used to

Fig. 4. The pathway to improve automatic analysis of sleep measurements with machine learning.

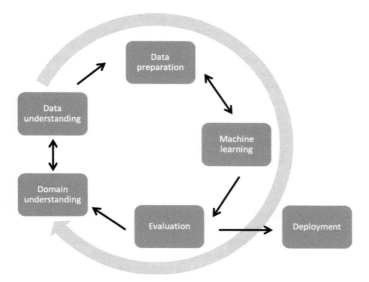

find similar patterns that can be used to describe common profiles of the observations in the data. Unsupervised learning is also used to detect anomalous observations that can be indications of errors in the data collection, or abnormal behavior that needs to be investigated further.[104] In sleep analysis, unsupervised learning can be used to find sleep patterns in the long-term data of 1 person or phenotypes in larger datasets as well as to, for example, identify sleep stages.[25,105–109] In contrast, supervised learning requires labeled data, such as events and class labels of the observations.[80] This approach is used to detect events during sleep, such as in OSA to discover intricate relationships between vital signs, events, sleep stages, and phenotypes, and predict future occurrences regarding health and well-being.[110–112]

Despite the vast amounts of available data of all types, the sleep research community has only recently started exploiting machine learning, and first results indicate their huge potential.[113] With the drastic advancement of technology and increase in computational power, a type of machine learning called deep learning has made a lasting mark in areas where complex, fine-grained, sequential data are in abundance, and the prevalence continues to grow.[114,115] Deep learning is a synonym for a variety of deep neural network architectures that are made up of several layers of artificial neurons that pass features of the input data between them while optimizing the importance of the links connecting the neurons in order to learn the structure in the data, either in an unsupervised or supervised manner.[116] In sleep research, deep neural networks have been trained on the various signals from a PSG to classify sleep stages, detect OSA, find distinction between people with and without specific symptoms, and predict sleep quality, to name a few.[117–119] Deep learning methods require massive datasets during training, but their unprecedented ability to discover patterns in highly complex data make them the prime contender to automatically analyze PSG data.

Limitations

A major limitation when performing supervised machine learning in traditional sleep studies is the need for labeled data. This labeling requires manual scoring by an expert somnologist or sleep technologist, where a sleep measurement is partitioned into sleep stages and various events are detected. It typically takes a trained sleep specialist 1.5 to 2 hours to score 1 overnight PSG and 30 minutes for a type 3 sleep study.[26]

Although efforts have been made to automate such scoring of sleep measurements,[120] the sleep specialist must still go over the whole recording afterward to edit the automatic scoring.[26,39]

Another limitation is the need for computational power, especially when working with deep neural networks. However, cloud solutions where models can be trained in reasonable time are becoming more readily available, which then may raise issues of data security, because the data are often sensitive. In addition, building deep neural networks with complex data requires expert knowledge and sufficient training, both on the technical side and in the domain where the data comes from. In the absence of such requirements, it will be necessary for sleep specialists to master the proper computer science knowledge to work with neural networks or for computer scientists to dive into the domain of sleep analysis. Collaboration between experts in the 2 fields is another way forward, which, in addition, fosters multidisciplinary research.

Future Potentials

There is a long tradition of using PSGs to diagnose sleep. However, PSGs are invasive and time consuming to analyze, as described earlier. Although PSG data are multivariate, complex, and of high frequency, they only provide a 1-night snapshot of the individual's sleep characteristics. In contrast, data from wearables offer fewer dimensions (heart rate, steps, sleep stages, and so forth), and the measurements are less frequent but they span a much longer time. Wearables are gaining popularity because they offer the possibility to track and analyze sleep and sleeping behavior for an extended period of time at an individual level. This ability can be seen as a single-subject (n = 1) clinical trial, where an individual patient is viewed as the sole unit of observation in the study. The goal is then to use data-driven methods to determine the optimal intervention for the individual.[121] Because the individual uses the wearables for a long time, it is possible to use the data collected to learn the individual's baseline behavior and then automatically detect patterns or observations that are out of the ordinary and could be signs of illness or cause for an intervention (ie, with a physician). The widespread use of wearables furthermore enables research on sleeping patterns and behaviors on larger and more heterogeneous cohorts of people than ever before. Recent studies confirm age-related changes in sleep as well as gender differences in sleep patterns.[122]

As mentioned earlier, there remains much research and development of deep learning methods to analyze sleep data. Current deep learning applications for sleep measurements build on convolutional neural networks and/or recurrent neural networks and have been shown to work well.[114] However, they are still limited by the scarcity of labeled data, for which active learning and transfer learning could offer a solution. In addition, reinforcement learning could be used in specific cases.

Active learning is an interactive machine learning scheme where the algorithm uses the available labeled data to train the model and then asks the expert using the system to label specific observations to enhance the learning and improve the model's performance.[123] This option would be especially useful for scoring sleep measurements, because the system could repeatedly query the expert for input, which leads to more labeled data, and perhaps provides the necessary distinction where the algorithm struggles, and it can thus focus its learning on the difficult gray areas. In this way, the algorithm actively learns from the expert.

Transfer learning is an approach where a deep learning model that is trained on a dataset in a specific domain is applied to another dataset in another domain. In the domain of sleep studies, there may be different devices that measure the same signals in slightly different ways.[124] As mentioned earlier, deep learning models require a lot of annotated and labeled data, which may not always be available. When many labeled data exist for 1 device, but not for another, it is possible to train a model to detect events using the richly annotated data, and then apply it to the other dataset even though it may be slightly different. This process is called transfer learning.

Reinforcement learning is a machine learning approach that learns optimal behavior by training an algorithm for a given task using trial and error to maximize the long-term reward.[112] It has not been applied in the sleep research community, to the best of our knowledge, but there is potential for it, for example, for personalization. Because data on sleep patterns are continuously collected through wearables, the algorithm that computes quality of sleep can be personalized using deep reinforcement learning. The approach would then accommodate individual patterns and behaviors and, over time, get better at assessing different sleep features at a personal level.

Data science offers much potential for the future of clinical practice, and for the future of sleep research, from gathering a wider variety of data to sophisticated modeling with deep learning architectures and insightful visualizations. This article goes through and suggests active learning, transfer learning, and reinforcement learning as concrete paths to take in machine learning with sleep data but also stresses the importance of developing new types of methods through sleep research as well as a focus on longitudinal data collected through wearables.

SUMMARY

This article argues for various ways of collecting data to enlighten the sleep research of the future. First, it describes the various types of subjective and objective data and discusses their limitations and future potential. Second, it highlights the prospects of digital management platforms to store and present the data, the importance of codesign when designing and developing such platforms, and the opportunities data science opens for the analysis of the data. Third, it shows the importance of considering data from different sources in the care of a patient, because it provides a means of seeing a fuller picture. Most of the data discussed in this article can be visualized for various stakeholder groups, through clever and insightful visualizations from which the health care professionals can draw informed decisions, and researchers can see trends from various sources, together in 1 visualization.

As the authors see it, the future of sleep research, and the future of informed clinical practice, is through the combination of various types of data. By introducing and combining new approaches from various research domains on the one hand and alongside patients and health care professionals on the other, clinicians will be able to understand new dimensions of the impact of sleep and lack of sleep that will affect and inform both research and clinical work for future improvements.

CLINICS CARE POINTS

- When performing a sleep assessment, do not rely only on objective sleep testing, because the subjective experience of the patient is equally important.
- Do not rely only on a single screening questionnaire to decide who needs further sleep testing, because most of these questionnaires are markedly flawed and validated in a limited way.

- Consider providing care via telemedicine where possible, such as with electronic questionnaires and sleep diaries.

- Be aware of the potential first-night effect of sleeping with a device, the night-to-night variability in different sleep parameters, and the limitations of different measurement types, which may affect clinical diagnosis. At present, manual scoring is still needed for sleep study analysis, and automatic analysis alone is not recommended for clinical use.

- At present, wearable and nonwearable data are not accepted for clinical use, and patients bringing such data to their health care personnel need to be educated about the limitations of these data.

ACKNOWLEDGMENTS

The authors thank Kristin Anna Ólafsdóttir, expert sleep technologist, and Dr Dirk Pevernagie for reviewing the article and providing excellent suggestions for improvements.

DISCLOSURE

Dr E.S. Arnardottir discloses lecture fees from Nox Medical, Philips, and ResMed. Dr A.S. Islind and Dr M. Óskarsdóttir have nothing to disclose. The work in this article is sponsored in part by the Sleep Revolution, which has received funding from the European Union's Horizon 2020 research and innovation program under grant agreement no. 965417 and by NordForsk (NordSleep project 90458-06111) via the Icelandic Centre for Research.

REFERENCES

1. Óskarsdóttir M, Bravo C, Sarraute C, et al. The value of big data for credit scoring: enhancing financial inclusion using mobile phone data and social network analytics. Appl Soft Comput 2019;74: 26–39.

2. Douglas JA, Chai-Coetzer CL, McEvoy D, et al. Guidelines for sleep studies in adults - a position statement of the Australasian Sleep Association. Sleep Med 2017;36(Suppl 1):S2–22.

3. International classification of sleep disorders. 3rd edition. Darien, IL: American Academy of Sleep Medicine; 2014.

4. Shahid A, Wilkinson K, Marcu S, et al. STOP, THAT and one hundred other sleep scales. Springer Science & Business Media; 2012.

5. Boynton G, Vahabzadeh A, Hammoud S, et al. Validation of the STOP-BANG questionnaire among patients referred for suspected obstructive sleep apnea. J Sleep Disord Treat Care 2013;2(4).

6. Silva GE, Vana KD, Goodwin JL, et al. Identification of patients with sleep disordered breathing: comparing the four-variable screening tool, STOP, STOP-Bang, and Epworth Sleepiness Scales. J Clin Sleep Med 2011;7(5):467–72.

7. Prasad KT, Sehgal IS, Agarwal R, et al. Assessing the likelihood of obstructive sleep apnea: a comparison of nine screening questionnaires. Sleep Breath 2017;21(4):909–17.

8. Hwang M, Zhang K, Nagappa M, et al. Validation of the STOP-Bang questionnaire as a screening tool for obstructive sleep apnoea in patients with cardiovascular risk factors: a systematic review and meta-analysis. BMJ Open Respir Res 2021;8(1): e000848.

9. Netzer NC, Stoohs RA, Netzer CM, et al. Using the Berlin Questionnaire to identify patients at risk for the sleep apnea syndrome. Ann Intern Med 1999; 131(7):485–91.

10. Marti-Soler H, Hirotsu C, Marques-Vidal P, et al. The NoSAS score for screening of sleep-disordered breathing: a derivation and validation study. Lancet Respir Med 2016;4(9):742–8.

11. Le Grande MR, Jackson AC, Beauchamp A, et al. Diagnostic accuracy and suitability of instruments that screen for obstructive sleep apnoea, insomnia and sleep quality in cardiac patients: a meta-analysis. Sleep Med 2021 :S1389-9457(21)00119-2.

12. Johns MW. A new method for measuring daytime sleepiness: the Epworth sleepiness scale. Sleep 1991;14(6):540–5.

13. Johns MW. Reliability and factor analysis of the Epworth sleepiness scale. Sleep 1992;15(4):376–81.

14. Johns MW. Daytime sleepiness, snoring, and obstructive sleep apnea. The Epworth Sleepiness Scale. Chest 1993;103(1):30–6.

15. Kaida K, Takahashi M, Akerstedt T, et al. Validation of the Karolinska sleepiness scale against performance and EEG variables. Clin Neurophysiol 2006;117(7):1574–81.

16. Hoddes E, Zarcone V, Smythe H, et al. Quantification of sleepiness: a new approach. Psychophysiology 1973;10(4):431–6.

17. Buysse DJ, Reynolds CF 3rd, Monk TH, et al. The Pittsburgh Sleep Quality Index: a new instrument for psychiatric practice and research. Psychiatry Res 1989;28(2):193–213.

18. Fedson AC, Pack AI, Gislason T. Frequently used sleep questionnaires in epidemiological and genetic research for obstructive sleep apnea: a review. Sleep Med Rev 2012;16(6):529–37.

19. Baldwin CM, Kapur VK, Holberg CJ, et al. Associations between gender and measures of daytime somnolence in the sleep heart health study. Sleep 2004;27(2):305–11.

20. Nigro CA, Dibur E, Borsini E, et al. The influence of gender on symptoms associated with obstructive sleep apnea. Sleep Breath 2018;22(3):683–93.

21. Bauters FA, Loof S, Hertegonne KB, et al. Sex-specific sleep apnea screening questionnaires: closing the performance gap in women. Sleep Med 2020;67:91–8.

22. Westbrook L, Saperstein A. New categories are not enough: rethinking the measurement of sex and gender in social surveys. Gend Soc 2015;29(4):534–60.

23. McNicholas WT. Screening for sleep-disordered breathing: the continuing search for a reliable predictive questionnaire. Lancet Respir Med 2016;4(9):683–5.

24. Tsang S, Royse CF, Terkawi AS. Guidelines for developing, translating, and validating a questionnaire in perioperative and pain medicine. Saudi J Anaesth 2017;11(Suppl 1):S80–9.

25. Keenan BT, Kim J, Singh B, et al. Recognizable clinical subtypes of obstructive sleep apnea across international sleep centers: a cluster analysis. Sleep 2018;41(3):zsx214.

26. Fischer J, Dogas Z, Bassetti CL, et al. Standard procedures for adults in accredited sleep medicine centres in Europe. J Sleep Res 2012;21(4):357–68.

27. Grote L, Puertas FJ. Assessment of sleep disorders and diagnostic procedures. 2. The clinical interview and clinical examination. In: Bassetti C, Dogas Z, Peigneux P, editors. Sleep medicine textbook. Regensburg: European Sleep Research Society; 2014. p. 111–23.

28. American Academy of Sleep Medicine. Available at: https://aasm.org/resources/medsleep/(harding) questions.pdf. Accessed March 15, 2021.

29. Merikangas KR, Zhang J, Emsellem H, et al. The structured diagnostic interview for sleep patterns and disorders: rationale and initial evaluation. Sleep Med 2014;15(5):530–5.

30. Taylor DJ, Wilkerson AK, Pruiksma KE, et al. Reliability of the structured clinical interview for DSM-5 sleep disorders module. J Clin Sleep Med 2018;14(3):459–64.

31. Boyatzis RE. Transforming qualitative information: thematic analysis and code development. Sage; 1998.

32. Guest G, MacQueen KM, Namey EE. Applied thematic analysis. Sage Publications; 2011.

33. Braun V, Clarke V. What can "thematic analysis" offer health and wellbeing researchers? Int J Qual Stud Health Well-being 2014;9:26152.

34. Buysse DJ, Ancoli-Israel S, Edinger JD, et al. Recommendations for a standard research assessment of insomnia. Sleep 2006;29(9):1155–73.

35. Morin CM. Measuring outcomes in randomized clinical trials of insomnia treatments. Sleep Med Rev 2003;7(3):263–79.

36. Carney CE, Buysse DJ, Ancoli-Israel S, et al. The consensus sleep diary: standardizing prospective sleep self-monitoring. Sleep 2012;35(2):287–302.

37. Riemann D, Baglioni C, Bassetti C, et al. European guideline for the diagnosis and treatment of insomnia. J Sleep Res 2017;26(6):675–700.

38. Palagini L, Manni R, Aguglia E, et al. Expert opinions and consensus recommendations for the evaluation and management of insomnia in clinical practice: joint statements of five Italian scientific societies. Front Psychiatry 2020;11:558.

39. Berry RB, Brooks R, Gamaldo CE, et al. The AASM manual for the scoring of sleep and associated events: rules, terminology and technical specifications, version 2.6. Darien, Illinois: American Academy of Sleep Medicine; 2020.

40. Kapur VK, Auckley DH, Chowdhuri S, et al. Clinical practice guideline for diagnostic testing for adult obstructive sleep apnea: an American Academy of Sleep Medicine clinical practice guideline. J Clin Sleep Med 2017;13(3):479–504.

41. Pevernagie DA, Gnidovec-Strazisar B, Grote L, et al. On the rise and fall of the apnea-hypopnea index: a historical review and critical appraisal. J Sleep Res 2020;29(4):e13066.

42. Arnardottir ES, Verbraecken J, Gonçalves M, et al. Variability in recording and scoring of respiratory events during sleep in Europe: a need for uniform standards. J Sleep Res 2016;25(2):144–57.

43. Chung F, Yang Y, Brown R, et al. Alternative scoring models of STOP-bang questionnaire improve specificity to detect undiagnosed obstructive sleep apnea. J Clin Sleep Med 2014;10(9):951–8.

44. Goldstein CA, Karnib H, Williams K, et al. The utility of home sleep apnea tests in patients with low versus high pre-test probability for moderate to severe OSA. Sleep Breath 2018;22(3):641–51.

45. Roeder M, Bradicich M, Schwarz EI, et al. Night-to-night variability of respiratory events in obstructive sleep apnoea: a systematic review and meta-analysis. Thorax 2020;75(12):1095–102.

46. Oksenberg A, Arons E, Nasser K, et al. REM-related obstructive sleep apnea: the effect of body position. J Clin Sleep Med 2010;6(4):343–8.

47. Gabryelska A, Białasiewicz P. Association between excessive daytime sleepiness, REM phenotype and severity of obstructive sleep apnea. Sci Rep 2020;10(1):1–6.

48. Srijithesh P, Aghoram R, Goel A, et al. Positional therapy for obstructive sleep apnoea. Cochrane Database Syst Rev 2019;(5):CD010990.

49. Andrade L, Paiva T. Ambulatory versus laboratory polysomnography in obstructive sleep apnea: comparative assessment of quality, clinical efficacy, treatment compliance, and quality of life. J Clin Sleep Med 2018;14(8):1323–31.

50. Zhang Z, Sowho M, Otvos T, et al. A comparison of automated and manual sleep staging and respiratory event recognition in a portable sleep diagnostic device with in-lab sleep study. J Clin Sleep Med 2020;16(4):563–73.

51. Dietz-Terjung S, Martin AR, Finnsson E, et al. Proof of principle study: diagnostic accuracy of a novel algorithm for the estimation of sleep stages and disease severity in patients with sleep-disordered breathing based on actigraphy and respiratory inductance plethysmography. Sleep Breath 2021.

52. Yalamanchali S, Farajian V, Hamilton C, et al. Diagnosis of obstructive sleep apnea by peripheral arterial tonometry: meta-analysis. JAMA Otolaryngol Head Neck Surg 2013;139(12):1343–50.

53. Maslow AH. The psychology of science. New York: Harper & Row; 1966.

54. Miettinen T, Myllymaa K, Westeren-Punnonen S, et al. Success rate and technical quality of home polysomnography with self-Applicable electrode set in subjects with possible sleep bruxism. IEEE J Biomed Health Inform 2018;22(4):1124–32.

55. Miettinen T, Myllymaa K, Muraja-Murro A, et al. Screen-printed ambulatory electrode set enables accurate diagnostics of sleep bruxism. J Sleep Res 2018;27(1):103–12.

56. Arnal PJ, Thorey V, Debellemaniere E, et al. The Dreem Headband compared to polysomnography for electroencephalographic signal acquisition and sleep staging. Sleep 2020;43(11):zsaa097.

57. Grote L, McNicholas WT, Hedner J, et al. Sleep apnoea management in Europe during the COVID-19 pandemic: data from the European sleep apnoea database (ESADA). Eur Respir J 2020;55(6): 2001323.

58. Korkalainen H, Leppanen T, Duce B, et al. Detailed assessment of sleep architecture with deep learning and shorter epoch-to-epoch duration reveals sleep fragmentation of patients with obstructive sleep apnea. IEEE J Biomed Health Inform 2020.

59. Randerath W, Bassetti CL, Bonsignore MR, et al. Challenges and perspectives in obstructive sleep apnoea: report by an ad hoc working group of the sleep disordered breathing group of the European respiratory society and the European sleep research society. Eur Respir J 2018;52(3):1702616.

60. Ancoli-Israel S, Martin JL, Blackwell T, et al. The SBSM guide to actigraphy monitoring: clinical and research applications. Behav Sleep Med 2015;13(sup1):S4–38.

61. Fekedulegn D, Andrew ME, Shi M, et al. Actigraphy-based assessment of sleep parameters. Ann Work Expo Health 2020;64(4):350–67.

62. Rognvaldsdottir V, Gudmundsdottir SL, Brychta RJ, et al. Sleep deficiency on school days in Icelandic youth, as assessed by wrist accelerometry. Sleep Med 2017;33:103–8.

63. Marino M, Li Y, Rueschman MN, et al. Measuring sleep: accuracy, sensitivity, and specificity of wrist actigraphy compared to polysomnography. Sleep 2013;36(11):1747–55.

64. Sadeh A, Acebo C. The role of actigraphy in sleep medicine. Sleep Med Rev 2002;6(2):113–24.

65. de Zambotti M, Godino JG, Baker FC, et al. The boom in wearable technology: cause for alarm or just what is needed to better understand sleep? Sleep 2016;39(9):1761–2.

66. Swan M. The quantified self: fundamental disruption in big data science and biological discovery. Big Data 2013;1(2):85–99.

67. Mettler T, Wulf J. Physiolytics at the workplace: affordances and constraints of wearables use from an employee's perspective. Inf Syst J 2019;29(1): 245–73.

68. Fox G, Connolly R. Mobile health technology adoption across generations: narrowing the digital divide. Inf Syst J 2018;28(6):995–1019.

69. Depner CM, Cheng PC, Devine JK, et al. Wearable technologies for developing sleep and circadian biomarkers: a summary of workshop discussions. Sleep 2020;43(2):zsz254.

70. Shelgikar AV, Anderson PF, Stephens MR. Sleep tracking, wearable technology, and opportunities for research and clinical care. Chest 2016;150(3): 732–43.

71. Ko P-RT, Kientz JA, Choe EK, et al. Consumer sleep technologies: a review of the landscape. J Clin Sleep Med 2015;11(12):1455–61.

72. de Zambotti M, Goldstone A, Claudatos S, et al. A validation study of Fitbit Charge 2 compared with polysomnography in adults. Chronobiol Int 2018;35(4):465–76.

73. Montgomery-Downs HE, Insana SP, Bond JA. Movement toward a novel activity monitoring device. Sleep Breath 2012;16(3):913–7.

74. Gruwez A, Libert W, Ameye L, et al. Reliability of commercially available sleep and activity trackers with manual switch-to-sleep mode activation in free-living healthy individuals. Int J Med Inform 2017;102:87–92.

75. Scott H, Lack L, Lovato N. A systematic review of the accuracy of sleep wearable devices for estimating sleep onset. Sleep Med Rev 2020;49:101227.

76. Baron KG, Duffecy J, Berendsen MA, et al. Feeling validated yet? A scoping review of the use of consumer-targeted wearable and mobile technology to measure and improve sleep. Sleep Med Rev 2018;40:151–9.

77. Evenson KR, Goto MM, Furberg RD. Systematic review of the validity and reliability of consumer-wearable activity trackers. Int J Behav Nutr Phys Activity 2015;12(1):1–22.

78. Kubala AG, Barone Gibbs B, Buysse DJ, et al. Field-based measurement of sleep: agreement

between six commercial activity monitors and a validated accelerometer. Behav Sleep Med 2020; 18(5):637–52.

79. Norström L, Islind AS, Lundh Snis UM. Algorithmic work: the impact of algorithms on work with social media. European Conference on Information Systems (ECIS) Research Papers; 2020. Available at : https://www.researchgate.net/publication/ 342421823_Algorithmic_Work_The_Impact_of_ Algorithms_on_Work_with_Social_Media.

80. Baron KG, Abbott S, Jao N, et al. Orthosomnia: are some patients taking the quantified self too far? J Clin Sleep Med 2017;13(2):351–4.

81. Bai Y, Hibbing P, Mantis C, et al. Comparative evaluation of heart rate-based monitors: apple watch vs fitbit charge HR. J Sports Sci 2018;36(15): 1734–41.

82. Li W, Bertisch SM, Mostofsky E, et al. Associations of daily weather and ambient air pollution with objectively assessed sleep duration and fragmentation: a prospective cohort study. Sleep Med 2020;75:181–7.

83. Cassol CM, Martinez D, da Silva FABS, et al. Is sleep apnea a winter disease?: meteorologic and sleep laboratory evidence collected over 1 decade. Chest 2012;142(6):1499–507.

84. Boe AJ, Koch LLM, O'Brien MK, et al. Automating sleep stage classification using wireless, wearable sensors. NPJ Digital Med 2019;2(1):131.

85. Islind AS, Lindroth T, Lundin J, et al. Co-designing a digital platform with boundary objects: bringing together heterogeneous users in healthcare. Health & Technology; 2019.

86. Islind AS. Platformization: co-designing digital platforms in practice. University West; 2018.

87. Bragazzi NL, Guglielmi O, Garbarino S. SleepOMICS: how big data can revolutionize sleep science. Int J Environ Res Public Health 2019;16(2):291.

88. Yoo Y, Henfridsson O, Lyytinen K. Research commentary—the new organizing logic of digital innovation: an agenda for information systems research. Inf Syst Res 2010;21(4):724–35.

89. Hylving L, Schultze U. Accomplishing the layered modular architecture in digital innovation: the case of the car's driver information module. The J Strateg Inf Syst 2020;29(3):101621.

90. Gawer A. Platforms, markets and innovation. Edward Elgar Publishing; 2011.

91. Ellingsen G, Monteiro E. Electronic patient record development in Norway: the case for an evolutionary strategy. Health Policy Technol 2012;1(1):16–21.

92. Fitzgerald G, Russo NL. The turnaround of the London ambulance service computer-aided despatch system (LASCAD). Eur J Inf Syst 2005;14(3):244–57.

93. Monteiro E, Pollock N, Hanseth O, et al. From artefacts to infrastructures. Comput Support Coop Work 2013;22(4–6):575–607.

94. Bødker S, Ehn P, Sjögren D, et al. Co-operative design—perspectives on 20 years with 'the scandinavian IT design model'. In: Proceedings from the proceedings of NordiCHI. Stockholm, October 23, 2000.

95. Islind AS, Lundh Snis U. From co-design to co-care: designing a collaborative practice in care. Syst Signs Actions 2018;11(1):1–24.

96. Sanders EB-N, Stappers PJ. Co-creation and the new landscapes of design. Co-design 2008;4(1): 5–18.

97. Cross N. Design research society conference. Design participation. London: Academy Editions; 1972.

98. Kensing F, Greenbaum J. Heritage: having a say. In: Routledge international handbook of participatory design. Routledge; 2013. p. 21–36.

99. Joshi SG, Bratteteig T. Designing for prolonged mastery. On involving old people in participatory design. Scand J Inf Syst 2016;28(1):1.

100. Woll A. Use of welfare technology in elderly care 2017. Available at: https://www.semanticscholar. org/paper/Use-of-Welfare-Technology-in-Elderly-Care-Woll/b9d2c252cb41a156ed6c9ed6f51513fe 3eba1b51.

101. Malmborg L, Binder T, Brandt E. Co-designing senior interaction: inspiration stories for participatory design with health and social care institutions. In: Proceedings from the workshop, PDC. Sydney, November 29 – December 3, 2010.

102. Baesens B. Analytics in a big data world: the essential guide to data science and its applications. Hokboken: John Wiley & Sons; 2014.

103. Shearer C. The CRISP-DM model: the new blueprint for data mining. J Data Warehousing 2000; 5(4):13–22.

104. Hastie T, Tibshirani R, Friedman J. The elements of statistical learning: data mining, inference, and prediction. New York: Springer Science & Business Media; 2009.

105. Zinchuk AV, Jeon S, Koo BB, et al. Polysomnographic phenotypes and their cardiovascular implications in obstructive sleep apnoea. Thorax 2018; 73(5):472–80.

106. Ma EY, Kim JW, Lee Y, et al. Combined unsupervised-supervised machine learning for phenotyping complex diseases with its application to obstructive sleep apnea. Sci Rep 2021;11(1): 4457.

107. El-Manzalawy Y, Buxton O, Honavar V. Sleep/wake state prediction and sleep parameter estimation using unsupervised classification via clustering. In: Proceedings from the 2017 IEEE international conference on bioinformatics and biomedicine (BIBM). Kansas City, November 13-16, 2017.

108. Pien GW, Ye L, Keenan BT, et al. Changing faces of obstructive sleep apnea: treatment effects by

cluster designation in the Icelandic sleep apnea cohort. Sleep 2018;41(3):zsx201.

109. Ye L, Pien GW, Ratcliffe SJ, et al. The different clinical faces of obstructive sleep apnoea: a cluster analysis. Eur Respir J 2014;44(6):1600–7.

110. Patti CR, Shahrbabaki SS, Dissanayaka C, et al. Application of random forest classifier for automatic sleep spindle detection. In: Proceedings from the 2015 IEEE biomedical circuits and systems conference (BioCAS). Atlanta, October 22-24, 2015.

111. Mendez MO, Ruini DD, Villantieri OP, et al. Detection of sleep apnea from surface ECG based on features extracted by an autoregressive model. In: Proceedings from the 2007 29th annual international conference of the IEEE engineering in medicine and biology society. Lyon, August 23-26, 2007.

112. Sutton RS, Barto AG. Reinforcement learning: an introduction. MIT Press; 2018.

113. Mostafa SS, Mendonça F, Ravelo-García AG, Morgado-Dias F. A systematic review of detecting sleep apnea using deep learning. Sensors 2019; 19(22):4934.

114. Fiorillo L, Puiatti A, Papandrea M, et al. Automated sleep scoring: a review of the latest approaches. Sleep Med Rev 2019;48:101204.

115. Gunnarsson BR, vanden Broucke S, Baesens B, et al. Deep learning for credit scoring: do or don't? Eur J Oper Res 2021;295(1):292–305.

116. Goodfellow I, Bengio Y, Courville A, et al. Deep learn, vol. 1. Cambridge: MIT Press Cambridge; 2016.

117. Zhai B, Perez-Pozuelo I, Clifton EA, et al. Making sense of sleep: multimodal sleep stage classification in a large, diverse population using movement and cardiac sensing. Proc ACM Interact Mob Wearable Ubiquitous Technol 2020;4(2):1–33.

118. Korkalainen H, Leppanen T, Aakko J, et al. Accurate deep learning-based sleep staging in a clinical population with suspected obstructive sleep apnea. IEEE J Biomed Health Inform 2019;24(7): 2073–81.

119. Korkalainen H, Aakko J, Duce B, et al. Deep learning enables sleep staging from photoplethysmogram for patients with suspected sleep apnea. Sleep 2020;43(11):zsaa098.

120. Penzel T, Conradt R. Computer based sleep recording and analysis. Sleep Med Rev 2000; 4(2):131–48.

121. Lillie EO, Patay B, Diamant J, et al. The n-of-1 clinical trial: the ultimate strategy for individualizing medicine? Per Med 2011;8(2):161–73.

122. Jonasdottir SS, Minor K, Lehmann S. Gender differences in nighttime sleep patterns and variability across the adult lifespan: a global-scale wearables study. Sleep 2021;44(2):zsaa169.

123. Settles B. Active learning. Synthesis lectures on artificial intelligence and machine learning. Morgan & Claypool Publishers 2012; 6: 1–114.

124. Torrey L, Shavlik J. Transfer learning. In: Olivas ES, Martin Guerrero JD, Sober MM, editors. Handbook of research on machine learning applications and trends: algorithms, methods, and techniques. IGI Global; 2010. p. 242–64.

Future Treatment of Sleep Disorders
Syndromic Approach Versus Management of Treatable Traits?

Dirk Pevernagie, MD, PhD[a,b,*]

KEYWORDS

- Sleep disorders • Sleep medicine • Obstructive sleep apnea • Endotype • Phenotype
- Precision medicine • Treatable trait • Fallacy

KEY POINTS

- Sleep medicine is cataloged according to a conventional disease classification system. Disease models are rooted in the pathophysiology of sleep. Polysomnography and other tests are used to demonstrate pathophysiological mechanisms underlying the currently known sleep disorders.
- Although many patients with sleep disorders may be adequately managed by this pathophysiological approach, therapeutic results are insufficient in some subjects, the causes of which lie in nonspecificity of symptoms, coincidental association between symptoms and pathophysiological endotype, as well as co-occurrence of two or more pathologic mechanisms affecting sleep.
- As co-occurrence of different pathogenetic mechanisms may produce phenotypes that are at odds with the idealized description of classic sleep disorders, the result of standard therapeutic interventions may be disappointing.
- The mechanisms underlying the expression of certain traits may be a substrate for targeted treatment. Treatable traits are characterized by biomarkers with predictive value as to beneficial treatment response.
- The challenge for the future is to gradually embrace the principles of systems medicine and to shift gear toward managing treatable traits in sleep disorders surpassing the limits of the traditional nosologic approach.

INTRODUCTION

Over the past decades, sleep medicine has evolved as a novel discipline in health care. The development of relevant medical specialties has invariably been preceded by major scientific advances in particular areas of interest. Medical and surgical specialties have traditionally been organized on anatomic or organ-based models in line with growing insight in organ-system physiology and pathology. The taxonomy of human disease dates back to the nineteenth century and is largely ascribed to the work of Sir William Osler, one of the founding fathers of modern medicine.[1] The classification of diseases by connecting the affected organ system with physiologic, anatomic, and histologic findings has been called the "Oslerian paradigm."[2] Syndromic patterns and nosologic entities are the building blocks of the Oslerian taxonomy that still prevails in the contemporary classification of human diseases.

Later in medical history, cross-sectional disciplines have emerged that are rooted in common

[a] Department of Respiratory Medicine, Ghent University Hospital, Corneel Heymanslaan 10, 9000 Gent, Belgium; [b] Department of Internal Medicine and Paediatrics, Faculty of Medicine and Health Sciences, Ghent University, Corneel Heymanslaan 10, 9000 Gent, Belgium
* Corresponding author.
E-mail address: dirk.pevernagie@ugent.be

Sleep Med Clin 16 (2021) 465–473
https://doi.org/10.1016/j.jsmc.2021.05.005
1556-407X/21/© 2021 The Author. Published by Elsevier Inc. This is an open access article under the CC BY-NC-ND license (http://creativecommons.org/licenses/by-nc-nd/4.0/).

biological settings and that integrate different organ systems in a particular context. Relevant "horizontal" disciplines have been developed in age domains (pediatrics and geriatrics), cell biology (oncology), microbiology (infectiology), to name a few. Sleep is an essential biological process that can be readily impaired by pathophysiological mechanisms. Evidently, the various sleep disorders have a common ground underpinning the concept of clinical sleep medicine as we know it today. The technological revolution over the past century has instigated sleep research, thereby disclosing a vast amount of scientific information and producing exquisite tools for diagnosing and treating sleep disorders. This evolution has paved the way for setting up sleep medicine as a medical discipline in its own right.[3] In line with this development, curricula in sleep medicine have been established uplifting it on a par with educational standards in other disciplines.[4]

In parallel with the creation of a professional title, textbooks, guidelines, and catalogs for disease classification have been published. The International Classification of Sleep Disorders (ICSD), issued by the American Academy of Sleep Medicine (AASM), is a concise reference book that systematically classifies the currently known disease entities of sleep.[5] In this manual, sleep disorders are categorized into various domains, including insomnia, sleep-disordered breathing, central hypersomnia, circadian rhythm disorders, parasomnia, sleep-related movement disorders, and miscellaneous conditions. The sleep disorders themselves are described by essential and associated features, predisposing and precipitating factors, natural course, pathophysiology, as well as results from polysomnography (PSG) and other objective tests. Basically, the items listed in the nosologic classification of the ICSD are modeled as disease entities. The disease model consists of a constellation of symptoms and signs complemented with characteristic pathophysiological findings on PSG (and other complementary tests). The merger of clinical findings and observations from diagnostic testing is deemed specific with respect to causality. The connotation of causality is reinforced by adding the term "syndrome" to certain disorders, for example, "sleep apnea syndrome" and "restless legs syndrome." Moreover, the ICSD provides diagnostic criteria for each nosologic entity. These criteria commonly include a mixture of symptoms, signs, and objective PSG findings. Diagnostic cutoffs are typically based on frequency and/or severity ratings of symptoms and PSG characteristics.

Inherently, a cause-consequence relationship is inferred for each sleep disorder listed in the ICSD,

the cause being a pathophysiological process demonstrable by PSG or other methods and the consequence being the clinical presentation. However, symptoms and signs overlap between nosologic entities and often correlate poorly with the degree of pathophysiological abnormality assessed by objective tests.[6] Not infrequently, the recommended therapy for sleep disorders fails to produce symptomatic relief or is not well tolerated, suggesting that the cause is not really affected by the treatment. In these cases, there are reasons to believe that causality is uncertain and that apparent or concealed confounders influence or determine the outcome. Thus, the question arises whether sleep medicine practice of the future should stick to the conventional "syndromic" approach or rather move to management of clinical traits that are likely to respond to targeted treatment?

Nosological Classification of Sleep Disorders: Evolution and Intrinsic Weaknesses

The AASM has revised the ICSD on several occasions. The nosologic classification of sleep disorders has been adjusted to integrate new scientific data. More emphasis has been placed on the role of pathophysiological observations on PSG. As a consequence, the theoretic concept of certain sleep disorders has evolved. To illustrate some conceptual adaptations over time, the present discussion will focus on the evolution of obstructive sleep apnea (OSA) as a model of chronic sleep disturbance across the consecutive editions of the ICSD, also highlighting some logical errors that inadvertently have crept in.

The first edition of the ICSD was published in 1990 by the American Sleep Disorders Association (the predecessor of the AASM).[7] The diagnostic criteria for OSA syndrome did not include any count of respiratory events nor the apnea-hypopnea index (AHI), but only a qualitative description: "frequent episodes of obstructed breathing." The severity criterion was primarily based on the seriousness of symptoms, which was assumed would be reflected in the PSG findings.

In 2005, The AASM published the second edition of the ICSD (ICSD-2).[8] The new version was at odds with the previous one in that AHI cutoff points were presented as the primary criterion for the definition of OSA. A diagnosis of OSA could be established based on an AHI greater than or equal to 5/h in the presence of symptoms or an AHI greater than or equal to 15/h even without symptoms. The cutoff points were inspired by an earlier AASM publication on OSA syndrome definition and measurement techniques.[9] In this paper, the AHI was introduced as a metric for gauging OSA severity. This proposition was based on a single cross-sectional population survey that showed an association between AHI and prevalent hypertension.[10] However, because this study did not include any prospective data at the time of publication, causal inference was scientifically inappropriate. Nevertheless, AHI was from then on accepted as the primary measure of OSA severity.

The AHI-driven remodeling of OSA has introduced a converse error (**Box 1**).[11,12] This error of reasoning reverses the logical order of premise and consequent: subjects with clinically relevant OSA have an increased AHI, but the converse is not necessarily true. The relevance of this error has become evident in epidemiologic research. In a Swiss survey on middle-aged to older people in an urban community, it was shown that the prevalence of an AHI greater than or equal to 15/h amounted to 49.7% in men and 23.4% in women.[13] In most of these people, daytime sleepiness or other symptoms of OSA were absent. Because an increased AHI can be demonstrated in large percentage of asymptomatic subjects in the general population, doubt must be casted on the validity of the AHI as meaningful metric of OSA disease severity.[6] Hence it follows that converse error will continue to distort the OSA disease model as long as the AHI is maintained as the prime predictor variable.

Box 1 also illustrates other deficiencies in reasoning related to false associations and assumptions.[11] In the ICSD-2, nosologic entities are described as sets of symptoms, signs, and PSG findings representing disease profiles with a common pathophysiological denominator. However, several sleep disorders have heterogeneous manifestations that do not simply fit a disease model cast into a concise set of diagnostic criteria. This reductionist approach may surely apply to certain subgroups, but by no means can it apply to all patients of the entire target group. Division fallacy is wrongly assuming that an individual belonging to a group (eg, subjects with an AHI $\geq$ 15/h) necessarily show other key characteristics of that group (eg, suffering from daytime sleepiness). It is often assumed that symptoms of OSA and increased AHI are causally related. Because this association can be due to coincidence, it is also a misconception. The quantitative (aka McNamara) fallacy is yet another misconception in which decisions rely solely on one metric, thereby ignoring all other observations.[14] The presumption that AHI by itself represents a disease state of OSA in a dose-dependent manner is not justified. The correlation between AHI and clinical manifestations is weak at best. Ascribing metric properties to the AHI is obviously an overqualification.[6]

The third edition of the ICSD (ICSD-3) has further expanded on OSA as a disease model, including mental, metabolic, and cardiovascular comorbidities as intrinsic components of the disorder.[15] Yet, no additional evidence was put forward in this edition to support the assumption that the AHI reflects clinical disease severity. Despite this omission, the ICSD-3 has been quoted as a reference for OSA severity rating in a recent clinical guideline on diagnostic testing of OSA published by the AASM.[16] The ICSD-3 takes the disease model even one step further, deleting the ultimate

---

Box 1
Logical relation between clinical presentation and increased apnea-hypopnea index in obstructive sleep apnea

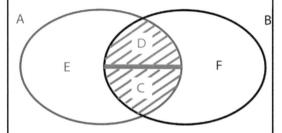

A: symptoms and signs that suggest OSA

B: increased AHI

C: causally related A and B (true positive)

D: coincidentally related A and B (false positive)

E: A with normal AHI

F: B without symptoms and signs that suggest OSA

Using B as a predictor for clinically relevant, treatment responsive OSA brings about fallacies:

Set B is a source of the McNamara or quantitative fallacy: AHI is a test result. Although it is commonly used as a metric of disease state, it misrepresents the clinical characteristics and severity of the disorder.

Set F is congruent with division fallacy: assuming that an increased AHI invariably represents symptomatic disease is erroneous. Many subjects are asymptomatic.

Sets C, D, and F are related to converse error (aka affirming the consequent): patients with true OSA (set C) have an increased AHI—the opposite is not necessarily true.

Set D represents association fallacy: false diagnosis of true OSA based on a coincidental association between A and B.

criterion described in IDSC-2 that "the disorder [ie OSA] is not better explained by another current sleep disorder, medical or neurologic disorder, medication use, or substance use disorder." The ICSD-3 clearly excludes the need for differential diagnosis and, as such, endorses association fallacy.

The aforementioned fallacies may have far-reaching consequences for clinical research and daily practice. There is as yet no gold standard (or "ground truth") to define the real disease state of OSA. The causative role of OSA in provoking symptoms and signs is hard to ascertain, even in the presence of high AHI values. As mentioned earlier, a coincidental association between an indicative clinical picture and increased AHI may be labeled as "false positive" OSA. In clinical practice, false-positively labeled patients with OSA will experience little benefit of therapy and may show poor adherence. Trying to optimize compliance to therapy in these individuals will not improve the clinical results. In clinical research, the outcomes of randomized controlled trials may be blurred by mixing up false-positive and true-positive OSA. The customary inclusion criterion of AHI greater than threshold will include both categories without knowing who's who. Obviously, the AHI bias will have to be addressed to improve future results in both clinical practice and research.[17]

New Perspective: Studying Heterogeneity and Complexity of Sleep Disorders

Chronic diseases are hallmarked by multicomponent and nonlinear pathologic processes and are ill-suited to be comprehended by reductionist models.[18] Instead, systems science offers tools to effectively treat susceptible traits at an individual level. Alvar Agusti has pioneered such approach in asthma and chronic obstructive pulmonary disease (COPD), two highly prevalent and disabling chronic diseases.[19] Taking obstructive lung disease as a starting point, he has elegantly described the historical transition of medical reasoning. Disease management, traditionally based on pathology- and pathophysiology-oriented diagnosis, had at some point to be fine-tuned. The first step was to identify differential disease attributes in patients with a common diagnosis allowing stratification into clinical phenotypes. However, such subclassification also proved insufficient to predict therapeutic effects and prognosis within the stratified subgroups. Eventually, it became obvious that a subsequent step had to be taken and that

assessment of disease characteristics was required at the individual level.[20]

At present, personalized (aka "precision") medicine is proposed as the ultimate paradigm to overcome the limitations of the former strategies. It is defined as "treatments targeted to the needs of individual patients on the basis of genetic, biomarker, phenotypic or psychosocial characteristics that distinguish a given patient from other patients with similar clinical presentations."[21] The main objective of precision medicine is to "improve clinical outcomes for individual patients while minimizing unnecessary side effects for those less likely to respond to a given treatment."[22] The rationale for assuming personalized medicine is the observation that chronic diseases are "complex" and "heterogeneous." In this setting, "complex" means that they have several components with nonlinear dynamic interactions, whereas "heterogeneous" indicates that not all of these components are present in all patients or, in a given patient, at all timepoints.[21] An explanation of these concepts is presented in **Table 1**.

The transition to personalized medicine is rooted in systems biology.[23] This scientific domain studies the complex time, space, and context-sensitive interactions of the vast amount of components that constitute a biological system. Information is lost by zooming in on the individual components. In order to gain new insights, the dynamics of the entire system must be analyzed at an integrated meta-level. Analytical methods are derived from systems engineering and big data science. The transposition of systems biology to the scientific domain of medicine is called "systems medicine" or "network medicine."[24] The intricate interaction of processes at environmental, clinical, biological, and genetic levels ultimately defines the clinical outcomes. In brief, the study of these complex mechanisms is grouped into basic domains covering genotypes, endotypes, and phenotypes (**Table 2**).[24] Meanwhile, the principles of precision medicine have been reviewed and deemed appropriate for common practice by opinion leaders of the sleep medicine community.[25,26]

Precision in Sleep Medicine

Endotypes and phenotypes have been studied intensively over the past decade, especially in the domain of sleep-disordered breathing.[27] An endotype denotes a particular mechanism that causes a physiologic or metabolic disturbance in certain organ systems. In OSA, several physiologic endotypes have been observed that, together, shape the disturbed breathing process. Members

Table 1
Evolution of the medical disease concept

Type of Disease Management	Underlying Concept	Clinical Implications	Management
Traditional medicine	Monodimensional, uniform disease processes	Syndromic approach: a common denominator of observed symptoms, signs, and pathologic markers defines the illness	"One size fits all"
Stratified medicine	Heterogeneity within nosologic entities	Phenotyping, stratification of subtypes	"One size fits every subtype"
Personalized medicine	Heterogeneity plus complexity within nosologic entities	Multiple causes or pathologic processes may underly discrete phenotypes. Discrimination between conventional nosologic entities becomes less obvious	Label-free, targeted therapy for treatment-responsive traits

Table 2
Definitions in systems medicine

Term	Meaning
Exposome	The cumulative/lifelong environmental exposures including smoking, pollution, noxious substances, infections, and diet.
Genome	The total composition of genes in a cell defining the genetic make-up of an organism or individual.
Epigenetics	Molecular mechanisms/multilevel biological networks that dynamically modulate the outcome of gene–environment interactions.
Genotype	The part of the genome (ie, a gene or set of genes) that codes for the characteristics of an organism or individual, determining the phenotype through the intermediary pathway of endotypes.
Endotype	The subtype of a condition that has a distinct molecular, functional, or pathobiological mechanism. Studying endotypes allows mechanistic approaches to disease stratification and treatment beyond the clinical presentation of the disease.
Phenotype	Observable characteristics of an organism or individual in health and disease. A combination of disease features, in relation to clinically meaningful attributes (symptoms, response to therapy, health outcomes, quality of life).
Trait	A particular characteristic such as an endotype or clinical subtype. A treatable trait is a therapeutic target identified by recognition of phenotype or endotype through validated biomarkers.
Biomarker	A measurable indicator (biological molecule in body fluids as well as physiologic phenomenon) used to gauge a particular biological or pathogenic process or response to treatment. Validated biomarkers may be reliable surrogates for certain endotypes or phenotypes.
Cluster	A set of characteristics that together point at a common cause or pathogenic mechanism

from the Division of Sleep Medicine at the Brigham and Women's Hospital (Harvard Medical School) have explored the pathophysiological mechanisms of sleep-disordered breathing.[28] Briefly, they demonstrated that several factors play a role in upper airway obstruction, including an anatomic feature predisposing to collapsibility of the upper airway, and nonanatomical traits (genioglossus muscle responsiveness, arousal threshold, and respiratory control stability—loop gain). In subsequent studies it was found that the nonanatomical pathophysiological traits are suitable to therapeutic options other than the conventional application of positive airway pressure therapy or the use of oral appliances.[29] More specifically, supplemental oxygen therapy or carboanhydrase inhibitors may be effective at reducing loop gain, whereas hypnotics may increase the arousal threshold, and upper airway muscle training or hypoglossal nerve stimulation may compensate for insufficient genioglossus muscle responsiveness.[27,30,31] Evidence is accumulating that physiologically targeted treatment of OSA may effectively decrease the AHI and thus lower the pathophysiological burden of the disorder. However, it is as yet uncertain whether this would also translate into reduced symptom scores.

Although the term "phenotype" can have different meanings, it usually denotes a combination of disease characteristics, in relation to clinically meaningful attributes (symptoms, treatment response, health outcomes, quality of life) that can be used to distinguish certain categories of patients from others.[32,33] Within taxonomically defined diseases such as OSA and COPD, the observed clinical heterogeneity necessitates subclassification into different clinical phenotypes. Cluster analysis is a suitable statistical method to discern subtypes in large heterogeneous groups. This technique has been explained in a recent review by Zinchuk and colleagues.[34] Cluster analysis uses hypothesis-generating (unsupervised) learning methods for discovering patterns in the parent population by grouping individuals into homogeneous categories, based on the clustering of particular features. The results depend on the parameters fed into the model and may focus on different outcomes including symptoms, PSG features, treatment results, and risk for having or developing comorbidities.

Cluster analysis has revealed remarkable findings in OSA research. Basically, three symptomatic forms of OSA have been identified, namely patients with disturbed sleep, minimal symptoms, and excessive sleepiness.[35] These observations have been replicated and expanded in a subsequent international, multicentric study.[36] In addition to the three basic clusters two other categories were proposed, that is, upper airway symptoms dominant and sleepiness dominant subtypes. Similar average AHI values were found in both study samples and across clusters, indicating that clinical phenotypes cannot be differentiated by the AHI. The disturbed sleep or "insomnia" phenotype was observed to be dominant in a survey of the European Sleep Apnoea Database.[37] In this study, phenotypes with insomnia symptoms comprised more than half of the patients with OSA and were more frequently linked with cardiovascular comorbidity than those with excessive sleepiness, despite less severe OSA. Using data from the Sleep Heart Health Study, the excessively sleepy subtype was found to be most strongly associated with prevalent heart failure and incident cardiovascular disease.[38] Cluster analysis of a multisite US Veteran cohort disclosed 7 OSA subtypes, when PSG data were fed into the statistical analysis.[39] In this study, certain physiologic endotypes (including those with periodic limb movement of sleep) captured risk of adverse cardiovascular outcomes, which was missed by the conventional AHI-based OSA severity classification.

Obviously, disparate results from cluster analyses regarding clinical phenotypes in OSA may reflect differences in patient samples and methods used. As yet, insufficient data exist to confirm that phenotypic clustering may be reproducible within the same datasets or across cohorts.[34] In accordance with other clinical trials, the target population for cluster analysis studies are subjects referred for OSA evaluation who happen to have an AHI greater than threshold. As previously explained, nonspecific symptoms such as insomnia or excessive sleepiness do not become specific markers of OSA in the presence of an increased AHI, and association fallacy may render the outcome of cluster analysis trials noninterpretable. The AHI should be considered the catch-22 of clinical OSA research. Addressing the "AHI bias" will be a major challenge for future clinical research.

Finally, OSA is not only complex and heterogeneous but also overlaps and co-occurs with other sleep disorders. Moreover, lifestyle characteristics and manifestations of medical and psychiatric comorbidities may further blend in with the palette of symptoms, thereby generating composed phenotypes. In order to predict responses to therapeutic interventions more reliably, unique mechanistic traits and clinical features of OSA will have to be determined.[27]

The Quest for Specificity: Discovering Markers that Indicate Treatable Traits

From the earlier discussion it becomes evident that the top-down Oslerian approach to disease, starting with the clinical presentation of the disorder at the top, followed by identifying the pathophysiological mechanisms below,[24] does not always work for sleep disorders medicine. In many patients with OSA the pathophysiological endotype does not seem to match the clinical phenotype.[27] The one-size-fits-all therapeutic strategies fail in a sizable number of patients categorized according to the prevailing ICSD. Cluster analysis has produced variable results and no consistent actionable information has come forth as to guide specific therapy in identified phenotypes. Furthermore, hypothesis-driven phenotyping is prone to circular reasoning, predisposing subjects to being labeled with the diagnostic outcome already before the diagnostic procedure has started (eg, "subjects referred for OSA evaluation"). Therefore, there is an opportunity for sleep medicine to leave the beaten path of Oslerian classification and to gradually adopt the principles of precision medicine.

To find markers that enhance specificity in the relationship between pathophysiological endotypes and the clinical phenotypes is a challenge of high priority. As clinical phenotypes in sleep medicine are often characterized by a set of nonspecific symptoms and signs, the identification of treatable traits is of prime importance. Traits can be considered as identifiers of causality between a pathogenetic mechanism and its clinical expression in the context of a disease model. The connotation "treatable" means that a trait may qualify as a decision aid for administering a targeted treatment that is expected to be effective. Treatable traits are not necessarily mutually exclusive. They can coexist in the same patient and can change with time.[24]

In OSA, the primary token of specificity regarding the relation between endotype and phenotype is a favorable response to therapy.[6] However, this is a post hoc finding of an ordinary trial-and-error approach, which is not quite appealing in the setting of modern medicine. The challenge is indeed to discover treatable traits that not only assure success of lowering the AHI but also, first and foremost, predict symptomatic response to targeted treatment. In recent years, investigators have sought to improve the diagnostic yield of clinical sleep studies. PSG offers exquisite multichannel and multivariable technology suited to demonstrate intricate pathophysiological mechanisms. It seems that routine PSG can be enhanced to emulate the (obtrusive and invasive) techniques that were used to validate the four endotypes described by Eckert and colleagues.[28,40,41] Furthermore, intelligent digital algorithms can be applied to expand the array of

PSG metrics, such as sleep depth, arousal characteristics, and hypoxic burden, among others.[42] The big data generated by thousands of polysomnographic recordings are an excellent substrate for novel analytical approaches. Innovative scoring techniques are expected to come out of the application of artificial intelligence. For example, hypnographic analysis of sleep has revealed a new sensitive and specific marker for type 1 narcolepsy, in the form of an unusual overlap between sleep stages.[43] Thus, innovation of PSG methodology holds promise for new biomarkers with a potential to serve as treatable traits.

The presence of soluble biomarkers in body fluids or exhaled air is another exciting field of scientific discovery. The study by Sànchez-de-la-Torre and colleagues was one of the first to show that biomarkers are capable of predicting treatment responses in patients susceptible to the hypertensive effects of OSA.[44] In this study, the presence of a particular microRNA profile was associated with the likelihood that blood pressure would be reduced by CPAP therapy in OSA patients with resistant hypertension. It can be expected that such information may assist in future decision-making regarding administration of CPAP versus prescribing antihypertensive drugs in this target group. In the domain of epigenetics, exploration of the transcriptome holds promise for the discovery of new biomarkers.[45] The noncoding RNAs, specifically microRNAs, seem relevant as potential indicators for the management of OSA, and the potential translational applicability of these molecules extends beyond predicting effects of CPAP on blood pressure.[45] Other potential biomarkers for OSA have been searched in the domain of proteomics.[46] Although some candidate markers have been identified, their accuracy is as yet insufficient to be implemented in clinical practice. Overall, the application of "-omics" seems promising for defining treatable traits, but the scientific development is still in its infancy. With the application of artificial intelligence and big data statistical analysis it is expected that useful biomarkers will emerge and will be integrated into clinical practice in the years to come.

In conclusion, it has become evident that the present nosologic classification of sleep disorders is too restricted. In the ICSD, sleep disorders have been parceled out into separate disease entities based on traditional taxonomy and pathophysiological modeling. In daily practice, however, nonspecificity of symptoms may confound diagnostic decision-making. Moreover, blended clinical conditions are frequently encountered for which clues as to choosing efficient and effective treatment are lacking. Therefore, it is time to downscale the Oslerian principle of disease management and to integrate systems medicine-based, unbiased ("label-free") approaches allowing effective treatment of traits that may be shared by different sleep disorders.

CLINICS CARE POINTS

- The treatment of sleep disorders is often straightforward, much to the satisfaction of the patient and the medical doctor. Patients presenting with complex phenotypes, however, may pose therapeutic problems.
- Treatment failure in clear-cut cases or problems in patients with complex phenomenology should prompt for other solutions than conventional therapy.
- The identification of traits that are responsive to targeted treatment is paramount in these cases.
- Although systems medicine—the driving force behind the development of personalized medicine—is at its infancy in the domain of sleep disorders, recent developments hold potential for diagnostic and therapeutic innovations that expectedly will become available for routine practice in the not-so-distant future.

DISCLOSURE

The author has nothing to disclose.

ACKNOWLEDGMENTS

This work has received funding from the European Union's Horizon 2020 research and innovation program under grant agreement No 965417.

REFERENCES

1. Loscalzo J, Barabasi AL. Systems biology and the future of medicine. Wiley Interdiscip Rev Syst Biol Med 2011;3(6):619–27.
2. Vanfleteren LE, Kocks JW, Stone IS, et al. Moving from the Oslerian paradigm to the post-genomic era: are asthma and COPD outdated terms? Thorax 2014;69(1):72–9.
3. Shepard JW Jr, Buysse DJ, Chesson AL Jr, et al. History of the development of sleep medicine in the United States. J Clin Sleep Med 2005;1(1):61–82.
4. Penzel T, Pevernagie D, Bassetti C, et al. Sleep medicine catalogue of knowledge and skills - Revision. J Sleep Res 2021;30(3):e13394.
5. Mayer G, Pevernagie D. Nosological classification and diagnostic strategy. In: Overeem S, Reading P, editors. Sleep disorders in neurology. A practical approach. 2 ed. Chichester, UK: Wiley-Blackwell; 2018. p. 41–52.
6. Pevernagie DA, Gnidovec-Strazisar B, Grote L, et al. On the rise and fall of the apnea-hypopnea index: a historical review and critical appraisal. J Sleep Res 2020;29(4):e13066.
7. ASDA. Obstructive sleep apnea syndrome (780.53-0). In: The international classification of sleep disorders - diagnostic and coding manual. 1 ed. Rochester, MN, USA: American Sleep Disorders Association; 1990. p. 52–8.
8. AASM. Obstructive sleep apnea, adult. In: Sateia M, Hauri P, editors. The international classification of sleep disorders - diagnostic and coding manual. 2 ed. Westchester, IL, USA: American Academy of Sleep Medicine; 2005. p. 51–5.
9. AASM. Sleep-related breathing disorders in adults: recommendations for syndrome definition and measurement techniques in clinical research. The Report of an American Academy of Sleep Medicine Task Force. Sleep 1999;22(5):667–89.
10. Young T, Peppard P, Palta M, et al. Population-based study of sleep-disordered breathing as a risk factor for hypertension. Arch Intern Med 1997;157(15):1746–52.
11. Damer TE. Attacking faulty reasoning. 6 ed. Belmont, USA: Wadsworth; 2009.
12. Heller J. Catch-22. London, UK: Vintage; 1994.
13. Heinzer R, Vat S, Marques-Vidal P, et al. Prevalence of sleep-disordered breathing in the general population: the HypnoLaus study. Lancet Respir Med 2015;3(4):310–8.
14. O'Mahony S. Medicine and the McNamara fallacy. J R Coll Physicians Edinb 2017;47(3):281–7.
15. AASM. Obstructive sleep apnea, adult. In: Sateia M, editor. The international classification of sleep disorders. 3 ed. Darien, IL, USA: American Academy of Sleep Medicine; 2014. p. 53–62.
16. Kapur VK, Auckley DH, Chowdhuri S, et al. Clinical practice guideline for diagnostic testing for adult obstructive sleep apnea: an American Academy of sleep medicine clinical practice guideline. J Clin Sleep Med 2017;13(3):479–504.
17. Randerath W, Bassetti CL, Bonsignore MR, et al. Challenges and perspectives in obstructive sleep apnoea: Report by an ad hoc working group of the sleep disordered breathing group of the European respiratory Society and the European sleep research Society. Eur Respir J 2018;52(3):1702616.
18. Ahn AC, Tewari M, Poon CS, et al. The limits of reductionism in medicine: could systems biology offer an alternative? Plos Med 2006;3(6):e208.

19. Agusti A, Bel E, Thomas M, et al. Treatable traits: toward precision medicine of chronic airway diseases. Eur Respir J 2016;47(2):410–9.

20. Agusti A. Phenotypes and disease characterization in chronic obstructive pulmonary disease. Toward the extinction of phenotypes? Ann Am Thorac Soc 2013;10(Suppl):S125–30.

21. Agusti A. The path to personalised medicine in COPD. Thorax 2014;69(9):857–64.

22. Jameson JL, Longo DL. Precision medicine–personalized, problematic, and promising. N Engl J Med 2015;372(23):2229–34.

23. Ahn AC, Tewari M, Poon CS, et al. The clinical applications of a systems approach. Plos Med 2006;3(7): e209.

24. Agusti A, Celli B, Faner R. What does endotyping mean for treatment in chronic obstructive pulmonary disease? Lancet 2017;390(10098):980–7.

25. Pack AI. Application of personalized, predictive, Preventative, and Participatory (P4) medicine to obstructive sleep apnea. A Roadmap for improving Care? Ann Am Thorac Soc 2016;13(9):1456–67.

26. Martinez-Garcia MA, Campos-Rodriguez F, Barbe F, et al. Precision medicine in obstructive sleep apnoea. Lancet Respir Med 2019;7(5):456–64.

27. Edwards BA, Redline S, Sands SA, et al. More than the Sum of the respiratory events: personalized medicine approaches for obstructive sleep apnea. Am J Respir Crit Care Med 2019;200(6):691–703.

28. Eckert DJ, White DP, Jordan AS, et al. Defining phenotypic causes of obstructive sleep apnea. Identification of novel therapeutic targets. Am J Respir Crit Care Med 2013;188(8):996–1004.

29. Carberry JC, Amatoury J, Eckert DJ. Personalized management approach for OSA. Chest 2018; 153(3):744–55.

30. Eckert DJ. Phenotypic approaches to obstructive sleep apnoea - new pathways for targeted therapy. Sleep Med Rev 2018;37:45–59.

31. Owens RL, Edwards BA, Eckert DJ, et al. An integrative model of physiological traits can be used to predict obstructive sleep apnea and response to non positive airway pressure therapy. Sleep 2015;38(6): 961–70.

32. Han MK, Agusti A, Calverley PM, et al. Chronic obstructive pulmonary disease phenotypes: the future of COPD. Am J Respir Crit Care Med 2010; 182(5):598–604.

33. Zinchuk AV, Gentry MJ, Concato J, et al. Phenotypes in obstructive sleep apnea: a definition, examples and evolution of approaches. Sleep Med Rev 2017;35:113–23.

34. Zinchuk A, Yaggi HK. Phenotypic subtypes of OSA: a challenge and opportunity for precision medicine. Chest 2020;157(2):403–20.

35. Ye L, Pien GW, Ratcliffe SJ, et al. The different clinical faces of obstructive sleep apnoea: a cluster analysis. Eur Respir J 2014;44(6):1600–7.

36. Keenan BT, Kim J, Singh B, et al. Recognizable clinical subtypes of obstructive sleep apnea across international sleep centers: a cluster analysis. Sleep 2018;41(3):zsx214.

37. Saaresranta T, Hedner J, Bonsignore MR, et al. Clinical phenotypes and comorbidity in European sleep apnoea patients. PLoS One 2016;11(10):e0163439.

38. Mazzotti DR, Keenan BT, Lim DC, et al. Symptom subtypes of obstructive sleep apnea predict incidence of cardiovascular outcomes. Am J Respir Crit Care Med 2019;200(4):493–506.

39. Zinchuk A, Yaggi HK. Sleep apnea heterogeneity, phenotypes, and cardiovascular risk. Implications for trial Design and precision sleep medicine. Am J Respir Crit Care Med 2019;200(4):412–3.

40. Sands SA, Edwards BA, Terrill PI, et al. Phenotyping Pharyngeal pathophysiology using polysomnography in patients with obstructive sleep apnea. Am J Respir Crit Care Med 2018;197(9):1187–97.

41. Bosi M, De Vito A, Kotecha B, et al. Phenotyping the pathophysiology of obstructive sleep apnea using polygraphy/polysomnography: a review of the literature. Sleep Breath 2018;22(3):579–92.

42. Lim DC, Mazzotti DR, Sutherland K, et al. Reinventing polysomnography in the age of precision medicine. Sleep Med Rev 2020;52:101313.

43. Stephansen JB, Olesen AN, Olsen M, et al. Neural network analysis of sleep stages enables efficient diagnosis of narcolepsy. Nat Commun 2018;9(1): 5229.

44. Sanchez-de-la-Torre M, Khalyfa A, Sanchez-de-la-Torre A, et al. Precision medicine in patients with resistant hypertension and obstructive sleep apnea: blood pressure response to continuous positive airway pressure treatment. J Am Coll Cardiol 2015; 66(9):1023–32.

45. Pinilla L, Barbe F, de Gonzalo-Calvo D. MicroRNAs to guide medical decision-making in obstructive sleep apnea: a review. Sleep Med Rev 2021;59: 101458.

46. De Luca Canto G, Pacheco-Pereira C, Aydinoz S, et al. Biomarkers associated with obstructive sleep apnea and morbidities: a scoping review. Sleep Med 2015;16(3):347–57.

New Trends and New Technologies in Sleep Medicine
Expanding Accessibility

Thomas Penzel, PhD*, Martin Glos, PhD, Ingo Fietze, MD, PhD

KEYWORDS

- Sleep research • Sleep medicine • Telemedicine • Smartphone apps • Wearables • Smartwatch
- Sleep apnea • Oximetry

KEY POINTS

- Automatic sleep stage analysis takes new strategies with hypnodensity plots and machine learning.
- Sensors for pulse wave and sound focus on new pathophysiology traits.
- New sensors implement contact-free sleep recording at home or elsewhere.
- Telemedicine in sleep medicine is used for data transmission and for improving patient management strategies.

INTRODUCTION

Sleep medicine as a clinical discipline evolved from sleep research. Sleep medicine is a young and interdisciplinary field in medicine. Knowledge has grown in parallel with technical developments. Sleep medicine has profited much from the introduction of digital technologies in medicine.

New technological developments are observed following the growth in knowledge in physiology, pathophysiology, diagnostic and therapeutic approaches, and management of sleep disorders. This article focuses on new technical developments in diagnostics and consequently on changes in the management of sleep disorders. Some new methodologies in diagnostic tools enable a better understanding of the physiology and pathophysiology of sleep disorders, leading to phenotyping of patients based on specific characteristics in diagnostic assessment. Several treatment approaches have been improved based on new technologies and some made possible by new technical developments.

From the beginning, sleep medicine took advantage of new technical developments. The technical advances in the area of diagnostics can be grouped into methods for sensor technologies; methods for the recording and analysis of sleep; methods for data transmission, specifically telemedicine; and methods for out-of-center and portable recording of sleep. All methods advanced much with digital technologies and computer-based support. As such, the big trend is that sleep medicine is going digital in terms of diagnosis, treatment, and management of patients. Going digital opens new challenges on data safety and data security and integration in electronic health records. These need to be addressed now.

AUTOMATED SLEEP SCORING

Already in the 1980s, computer-based recording and analysis of recorded signals were probed in sleep laboratories. A paper-based sleep recording was limited to the way it was written on paper. No change of view on the signals (changing amplitude or time resolution) was possible. No copy of the recording (besides a paper copy) was possible. An archiving, an exchange of sleep recordings, was possible only with the paper sleep

Charité Universitätsmedizin Berlin, Interdisciplinary Sleep Medicine Center, Charitéplatz 1, Berlin 10117, Germany
* Corresponding author.
E-mail address: Thomas.penzel@charite.de

Sleep Med Clin 16 (2021) 475–483
https://doi.org/10.1016/j.jsmc.2021.05.010
1556-407X/21/© 2021 Elsevier Inc. All rights reserved.

electroencephalogram (EEG) books. Digital recording of sleep recordings immediately solved this set of problems. And immediately first steps were taken to develop computer assisted sleep analyses to derive abbreviated information and diagnosis from the large amount of recorded data. The recording no longer is a single document but can be reproduced or copied without quality loss. The recording can be viewed on different machines, with different monitors taking advantage of modified amplitude and time scale settings. Visual scoring by a technologist can be repeated at a different machine at a different location and at a different time. With having digital sleep recordings, it easily was possible to compare the visual sleep signal scoring between different sleep scorers and check agreement and discuss different interpretations. Checking of reliability of sleep scoring became possible and reliability of sleep scoring increased immediately. Training of sleep scoring could be done anywhere and independent of special sleep recording equipment. Visual scoring rules, such as those by Rechtschaffen and Kales,[1] became reproducible and universal. Based on the rules by Rechtschaffen and Kales results on sleep reports became reliable and easily comparable. Several studies did show a sufficient reliability, even if a lot of criticism remained.[2] With additional recommendation for the digital recording and the selection of signals for sleep recording in addition to the scoring rules, the basis for a uniform sleep recording was set.[3] The rules for visual scoring were simplified in many aspects in order to increase reliability and reduce inter-scorer and intra-scorer variability. Another aim for making the rules more reliable and having them described with more detail and precision was to facilitate the development of rule based automated algorithms for computer-assisted sleep staging in the future.[4] Definite recommendation and rules for an automated sleep stage analysis, however, were not consented. Instead, many engineering-based research groups still try to achieve an excellent computer supported sleep staging and present validation studies with improved results.[5] In parallel with the development of visual analysis of sleep scoring, sleep researchers have tried to develop data-driven sleep staging, not bound to the visual interpretation of human scorers. This approach is analyzing the sleep EEG signal, electrooculogram (EOG), and electromyogram (EMG) signal in order to derive sleep stages by the calculation of new metrics. One popular parameter is the odds ratio product of sleep-EEG, which can be regarded as a measure for the synchronicity of sleep.[6] More recent methods make use of increased computational power and apply new methodologies like machine learning and new neural network and artificial intelligence algorithms.[7,8] The aim always is to derive parameters that describe how deep sleep is, how sleep disruption and sleep fragmentation can be described, independent of discrete sleep stages and independent of arbitrary 30-second epochs as established for visual sleep scoring. The new methods use all kinds of algorithms, such as the ones discussed (artificial intelligence, artificial neural networks, big data analysis, and machine learning algorithms). Typically, some features need to be identified, which have been described visually, such as alpha, theta, and delta waves; sleep spindles; K-complexes; and arousals. In the end, usually a validation for the new method is used. An important limitation in the development of new methods needs to be considered. Often, a validation against the old visual sleep staging is requested. Studies usually perform validations against Rechtschaffen and Kales[1] or American Academy of Sleep Medicine rules.[4] New methods, overcoming the old visual sleep staging, will fulfill the expectations on validity and agreement only partially. If a new validation is performed, then the question is to validate against which truth. It would be optimal to find ground truth measure of the deepness of sleep or of memory consolidation during sleep. Increasingly it was recognized that there is a difficulty in general finding the ground truth for sleep recreation functions. As a consequence, developers of automatic algorithms chose the simple path and tried to imitate the visual scoring. The limitations to make this imitation perfect also are inherent to visual scoring. There always will be an inter-scorer and an intra-scorer variability.

A totally different approach, then, is to assume that all scorers are correct and that their scoring is seen as a probability to the correct classification of a certain sleep EEG epoch. This kind of probability-based sleep scoring recently has been used to develop a new automated scoring using big data analysis. To compare the results of the big data analysis sleep scoring against visual scoring, probabilities were calculated for each single sleep EEG epoch. This new probability-based sleep profile is called a hypnodensity plot for sleep stages.[9] Based on probabilities, this reflects the opinion of 8 or more sleep scorers on a certain sleep epoch. This is then applicable for the complete course of the night. This is useful, especially when applied to sleep scoring in patients with disorders of sleep regulation, such as narcolepsy. The developer does not need to negotiate with the visual scorer whether the scoring of a certain epoch may be erroneous but simply looks at the probabilities of several scorers for this epoch.

In summary, it is assumed that there are 2 possible future approaches for automatic sleep scoring. One is based on probabilities using many visual sleep scorers and sums up their results as probabilities for sleep EEG epochs. The other approach aims for a ground truth of sleep; however, for that, identifying new correlates for the functions of sleep is needed first.

SENSOR AND DEVICE DEVELOPMENT

Sensors used with polysomnography are used to record electrophysiologic signals generated by the body and several other signals that need to be converted into electrical signals. Directly recorded electrophysiologic signals are the EEG, EOG, and EMG of a few facial muscles and a few muscles in the periphery, typically the legs. The electrocardiogram (ECG) is the electrophysiologic sign that was recorded for the longest time, due to its strength in terms of voltage. Signals recorded during sleep, which require transducers, are respiratory, cardiovascular, and other indirect signals. Respiration is recorded in terms of airflow at the nose and mouth. Airflow can be picked up by thermosensitive sensors (thermistor or thermocouple) and by pressure sensitive sensors (nasal cannula). Respiration needs to be recorded in addition as respiratory effort. Respiratory effort can be recorded as the esophageal pressure generated by the respiratory muscles during inspiration. Alternatively, it can be recorded as movements of ribcage and abdomen. These movements are sensed by different types of belt. Piezoelectric sensors were popular for a long period due to their simplicity and low cost. Because they do not correlate well with the effective volume changes in the thorax, however, the method recommended today is inductive plethysmography. This method allows to estimate volume changes of the thorax because the signal is proportional to the cross sectional area inside the belt. The effect of respiration is reflected by blood gas changes, first of all oxygen saturation and carbon dioxide (CO_2) concentration. Oxygen saturation now is derived from a pulse oximeter, typically attached to a finger of the person. This signal requires a lot of signal processing from recorded pulse waves. CO_2 can be recorded transcutaneous as partial pressure with a sensor on the skin or as end-tidal CO_2 concentration in the exhaled air. Additional signals are body position, noise in the room, noise recorded with a body-worn microphone (both for snoring), and behavior with a video camera. Polysomnography

often allows to record additional signals like pulse wave, blood pressure, ventilated pressure (delivered by a positive airway pressure [PAP] therapy to the patient), esophageal pressure, esophageal pH, and core or skin body temperature. All of these classic sensors require electrodes or transducers, then signal filtering, digitalization, and recording with optimal resolution in time and in amplitude. All these sensors require cables and leads. New sensors try to reduce the number of leads or try to gain more information from just 1 signal or try to pick up signals contact-free. This is done to make the sleep recording more comfortable and to gain more information from fewer sensors. In addition, developers wish to derive additional physiologic information about sleep processes from the new sensors, which was not recorded before. With this, the hope is to gain additional insight in physiologic functions during sleep.[10]

Wireless transmission of physiologic signals recorded at the body is possible using modern wireless signal transmission technologies like Zigbee, Bluetooth, and similar short-distance transmission protocols. In the meantime, wireless signal transmission technologies are popular in new polysomnographic systems in order to reduce the cables between the body and a recording unit. This network of sensors and body worn modules is called a body area network.

Wireless monitoring of sleep has also advanced from early sensors to new modern applications. One early wireless sensor was a movement sensing foil placed in the bed underneath the sleeping person. Sensing devices in this category were presented by research groups from Finland—called static charge sensitive bed.[11] These devices used different kinds of electronic pressure sensitive foils for sleep and respiration recording. These foils became popular for the detection of sudden infant death syndrome. For that purpose the unit was connected with an alarm giving processing unit. The signal is called a ballistocardiogram (BCG). The BCG signal was filtered into 3 components reflecting heart rate, respiration, and major movements. For the first sensor devices, the splitting into the 3 components was achieved with analog bandpass filters separating the components according to different main frequency bands. With digital processing, an improved separation of the 3 components was possible, because it is obvious that there is considerable frequency overlap between the components characteristic for heartbeat, respiration, and coarse movements. Advanced sensor foils not only generated 1 signal from the sleeping subject but also used a field of sensors, possibly up to 144 sensor fields, into which the foil was divided, each giving the 3 components. Extensive computational power was needed for the many signal generating fields. This large amount of data allowed to derive better correlates for heart rate, respiration, and movements. By comparing the different fields, it was possible to derive body position of the sleeping person as well. Paalasma and colleagues[12] used a less costly approach and shrunk the sensor again, coming to a strip, which could be placed in bed underneath the blanket. This strip then was connected to a smartphone app and could provide information about wake, light sleep, deep sleep, respiration, and respiratory events. This strip now is sold by a smartphone app store as a consumer-oriented self-quantifying device, even if the underlying sensor technology is sophisticated and the analysis software validated extensively in a sleep center.

The next technological step was to make a distant recording of body movements by radar technologies. Radar or microwave radiation can pick up very small distance movements as generated on the chest wall by the heartbeat and by respiration. Microwaves pass through linen and duvets and thereby record an equivalent of the BCG from a distance. Again, heartbeat-generated movement, respiration, and coarse movements can be derived from a compound radar-based signal. The generating and sensing device can be placed near the bed. Similar to BCG, signal analysis can derive wake, light sleep, deep sleep, heart rate, and sleep-disordered breathing with a good signal analysis algorithm.[13] Such contact-free recording of sleep and sleep disorders now can be used outside of sleep centers, such as in any hospital ward, other hospitals without sleep laboratory service, nursing homes, or any home environment. Sleep recording can be done anywhere outside the controlled setting of the sleep center. This needs to be considered, because bedroom noise, ambient light, temperature, nutrition habits also are out of control.

The sensor technology inside a sleep center also profited from the development in medical technology over the past years. Pulse wave now often is recorded in parallel with oximetry sensors. The pulse wave signal is part of any pulse oximetry and was not recorded in the past. The analysis of the pulse wave signal allows calculating pulse frequency. A portable system often records pulse frequency instead of ECG-derived heart rate. If both are recorded, pulse wave and ECG, then it is possible to calculate the time between the electrical activity of the heart and the arrival time of the pulse wave in the periphery. This time is called pulse transit time (PTT). PTT is determined by many factors; some of them vary in short time spans. One such varying component is blood vessel compliance. Blood vessel compliance is related inversely to blood pressure. Therefore, PTT can be used to estimate blood pressure beat-to-beat continuously under the condition that a point calibration against sphygmomanometer-determined blood pressure (traditional arm cuff measurement) is performed at the beginning and the end of the signal recording. A recent validation study showed reasonably good correlation of the estimated relative blood pressure changes with other more established noninvasive continuous methods, such as finger plethysmography.[14] The more established finger plethysmography (Finapres [Ohmeda, Boulder Colorado] and Portapres [TNO, Amsterdam, The Netherlands]) is an expensive method, which performs a pressure clamping of the finger, so that transmural pressure is set to zero; thus, it is relatively uncomfortable and disturbs sleep in the subject who is investigated. Consequently, this method is not used widely but only in specific research studies.

An analysis of other characteristics of the pulse wave reflects the cardiovascular risk of patients. Based on this concept, an autonomic state index was introduced validated against the risk score for cardiovascular risk as established by the European Society of Cardiology/European Society of Hypertension. Using this new autonomic state index, it is possible to derive a cardiovascular risk by the recording and analysis of the pulse waveform alone.[15] This risk score assessment is of particular importance for patients with sleep-disordered breathing in order to support the treatment decision (Somnocheck micro cardio, Löwenstein Medical, Bad Ems, Germany).

More parameters can be extracted from the pulse waveform. These can parameterize the slope of the rise of pulse wave after each heartbeat and the reflection of the pulse wave in the artery (Windkessel reflection) in order to improve estimation of derived signals. A system that exploits a specially treated pulse waveform is the WatchPAT system (Itamar Medical Ltd, Cesarea, Israel), which records and analyses an attenuated finger pulse wave, called peripheral arterial tonometry.[16] Because the signal reflects sympathetic tone in the periphery it can be used to detect light sleep, deep sleep, and rapid eye movement (REM) sleep just from signal processing of the pulse wave amplitude and pulse wave rhythmicity.[17] Combined with a pulse oximetry sensor and a wrist-worn actigraphy, the recording and analysis boiled down to a portable system for the diagnosis of sleep-disordered breathing. Multiple validation studies showed accuracy versus polysomnography in detecting sleep stages in a coarse way and detecting respiratory events.[18] A recent publication showed the possibility of distinguishing central and obstructive apnea events.[19] With this large number of studies, this system produced enough evidence to be included in guidelines for the diagnosis of sleep disordered breathing.

The development of dedicated microphones for snoring become another subject of continuous improvement. Not only can the microphone record snoring, but also can the signal be divided into different frequency components, which allows distinguishing breathing, snoring, and movement artifacts.[20] Recent studies with a new sensor which combines a microphone and a pressure sensor, the Pneavox sensor (CIDELEC, St. Gemmes sur Loire, France) performed a validation study against polysomnography combined with esophageal pressure.[21] This more sophisticated recording and analysis allows distinguishing central and obstructive sleep apnea events, which is of importance for a decision on subsequent therapy for these patients.

HOME SLEEP TESTING REPLACES POLYSOMNOGRAPHY

The portable recording of sleep for the diagnosis of sleep apnea—polygraphy—is well established in many countries worldwide. Devices typically are national products and well validated and usually are accepted by the national reimbursement systems as diagnostic tools for the diagnosis of sleep apnea without comorbidities.[22] This diagnostic procedure usually is consolidated by national guidelines and recommendations.[23]

There is a need to classify devices for home sleep apnea testing. Initially, the number of signals or channels were counted. Recording systems were classified based on this simple number.[24] The classification defined level I systems as able to record 7 or more signals together with human supervision (eg, polysomnography), level II as systems again with 7 channels but without supervision (eg, home-based polysomnography), level III as systems with at least 4 channels (eg, polygraphy for sleep apnea), and level IV as systems with fewer than 4 channels (eg, pulse oximetry).[24] A newer and much more appropriate system is based on the physiologic information needed to achieve a sufficient diagnosis.[25] For obtaining information about sleep, cardiovascular system, respiration, and body position, a scoring system called SCOPER was developed and presented.[25] SCOPER is an acronym for sleep, cardiovascular, oxygen, position, effort (respiratory), and

respiration (airflow). For each of these information domains, a direct and optimal method is defined. For sleep, this is a 3-lead EEG. Lower-quality levels are defined as well, such as a 1-lead EEG signal, or actigraphy, or even more indirect signals, such as estimation of sleep derived from other signals. This kind of quality grading is defined for each of the 5 information domains. This grading system allows a categorization of out-of-center recording devices, such as polygraphy devices. Moreover, this grading system paves the way for an indirect assessment of sleep disorders, as can be done by smartphones and smartwatches. A smartwatch may be able to record oximetry perfectly. For the domain of oximetry the smartwatch reaches high quality. The pulse wave, going along with the oximetry, may be analyzed with good algorithms and these derive sleep stages. This is a low-quality grade for sleep stages due to the indirect nature of the measurement. Still, the indirect measurement has its justification and may prove quality with validation studies. The SCOPER system frees the user from counting channels, because this no longer is appropriate when algorithms extract multiple information out of a complex and digitally treated signal.

Modern smartphones offer multiple health apps as part of their regular preinstalled app collection. Many of these health apps allow estimating sleep and wake based on activity recording derived from the built-in 3-axis accelerometer in mobile phones. Often the algorithms are based on early research results derived from previously published actimetry algorithms.[26] Some apps integrate further user activity from the smartphone owner in order to improve the estimation of sleep and wake. This can be the local time, light recordings from the camera, and the owner using the smartphone.[27] Smartwatches or wrist-worn wearables often have additional optical sensors to record the pulse wave and derive pulse frequency and oximetry (**Fig. 1**). Pulse wave amplitude varies with respiration and sleep stages and might be used to improve an estimate of sleep classification. Based on more sophisticated algorithms, some apps estimate phases of light sleep, deep sleep, and REM sleep, based on the same physiologic principles described previously. Some wearables may be able to detect sleep-disordered breathing and may report apnea events in addition to sleep classification.[28]

Only a few health apps with sleep monitoring capabilities, however, have been validated against polysomnography in a sleep center. Usually the smartphone companies do not want to invest in expensive validation studies of adequate size and do not want to pick up the challenge of

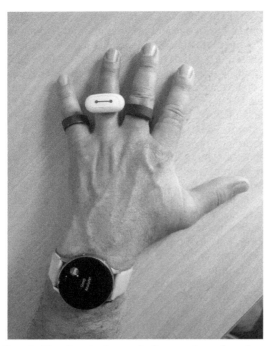

Fig. 1. The hand shows 3 finger rings for sleep recording and a smartwatch. The finger rings from left to right are Oura (Oura Health Ltd, Oulu, Finland), Sleepon (China), and Circul (Bodimetrics, China). The rings and the smartwatch have integrated pulse oximetry and activity monitoring to estimate sleep stages and sleep apnea events.

medical device certification. Medical software does require medical device certification if used to provide diagnostic information or advice. Often, companies are satisfied with providing consumer technology apps for self-quantifying or for gamification of health issues. This background of development approaches causes a wide range of accuracy and reliability in sleep apps available.[29] It is almost impossible to predict whether a certain app was developed in a joint enterprise with a sleep laboratory and was extensively validated or whether the app was developed by engineers reading some publications and testing the recording on a few test sets. Some apps are extremely good and accurate for detecting sleep stages and for detecting sleep apnea, even if they do not claim to be so reliable and even if they are not marketed as medical certified software. In that case, not obtaining the medical device approval may be a marketing decision of the company.

As a summarizing result for clinical use, it currently is impossible to trust sleep apps. As a sleep physician, the information should not be underestimated and can be a complement to the report and complaints of a patient. The app results

may be used to initiate regular sleep testing with validated technology. If a sleep app used by a patient appears to have some validity, possibly in a patient with insomnia, then it may be possible to recommend further use by the patient.

With the increasing digitalization of sleep medicine, a new class of sleep apps has been developed and become popular. These apps support electronic cognitive behavior therapy for insomnia patients. These apps may help patients communicate with their physician and follow behavioral advice to lower stress and follow the rules of sleep hygiene, as taught by psychologists and sleep physicians regularly. Currently, these apps are evaluated by sleep laboratories together with health insurances to estimate their effect on health care costs under the assumption that this kind of interaction may be beneficial in terms of insomnia and individual costs consuming health care resources.[30]

Another family of apps used in sleep medicine logs usage activities of a PAP therapy device in patients with sleep apnea. A patient with sleep apnea who is a user of an automated PAP, bilevel PAP, or continuous PAP device can check the time the device was used overnight. Because the PAP machines record airflow and leakage, they can report residual apnea and hypopnea events and they can record problems with leakage and with the mask used with the machine. These details are accessible to the patient using the appropriate app provided by the manufacturer. The app then may provide tips and recommendations to the user on how to deal with problems with the mask or if a consultation of the sleep physician is needed. The adherence monitoring app also may transmit these data to a service provider responsible for the PAP device, if the patient agrees and if national regulations support this kind of patient therapy adherence monitoring. Some countries, such as France, even require this electronic patient adherence monitoring in order to intervene early if therapy adherence drops below a certain threshold. Then, the service provider is asked to help the patient to overcome problems or to consult a sleep physician if a change in PAP ventilation is needed or if other changes like weight gain or upcoming comorbidities require treatment changes. An anonymous evaluation of PAP usage data reveals common and less common patterns of use, which enable options to improve long-term therapy adherence with individually tailored tips and counseling.[31]

Taken together, the developments of wearables and smartphone apps are valuable in the area of sleep medicine. They offer many possibilities, because everybody has sleep that is more or less healthy. They can be helpful in sleep disorders, because most sleep disorders are chronic disorders and require long-term therapy. In order to grade sleep apps when results are presented to a sleep physician, it would be helpful to introduce a certification system that offers trust in reliability and accuracy of the information provided. With such a system, it could be possible to distinguish sleep apps that are useful for sleep medicine versus those that are more for consumer satisfaction. The next step would be that sleep apps with useful medical information could share their results with electronic health care records using a certified medical data interchange mechanism. Then, the recorded data could become useful for sleep physicians as well. It may require some more time to develop the corresponding security protocols for safe and secure data transmission. Finally, the new security and safety protocols can provide improved patient care and transparency to patients suffering from sleep disorders.

The importance and the role of sleep laboratory–based polysomnography will change. It still will be used as a clinical research tool and a reference when validating new devices for some kind of sleep recording.[32] In some countries, home-based polysomnography has become popular. In other countries, polysomnography has decreased and been replaced by polygraphy or home sleep apnea testing. There still are many countries that do not have enough sleep medicine service and in these countries simpler tools, such as polygraphy or a few channel-based systems, like portable oximetry, play another role compared with more developed countries. The development of wearables and sleep apps may help in this area, however, only if these are certified and fulfill certain minimal criteria on accuracy and reliability. Otherwise, those wearables and sleep apps need to remain in the arena of consumer tools and lifestyle apps.

TELEMEDICINE APPLICATION IN MANAGEMENT OF SLEEP MEDICINE

Telemedicine in sleep medicine covers a broad area of applications and options.[33] In general, these cover diagnostic tools, therapy support tools, patient management, medical appointment management, transmission of medical results and reports, continuous monitoring of therapy, video consultation, and video counseling.

Within the discipline of sleep medicine, the term' telemedicine, usually is associated with the monitoring of adherence to PAP therapy in patients with sleep apnea (see Johan Verbraecken's article, "Telemedicine in Sleep-Disordered Breathing: Expanding the Horizons," in this issue.). This is a telemedicine application. It is discussed previously, and it presents only a small and specialized app–linked aspect of telemedicine. Within sleep medicine, there are many more telemedicine applications. The telemonitoring of PAP compliance can be simple. It can be implemented as just a text message sent by the PAP machine to the service provider, giving the therapy usage time. It can contain a large amount of data, including flow curves and leakage signals, to allow an analysis of the curves and provide a diagnosis on residual respiratory events during the previous night and a detection of problems with therapy. The telemonitoring costs are paid by health insurance in some countries because this supervision and the linked service increases PAP usage and thereby effective treatment. The information transmission can be not only from the machine to the service provider but also in the opposite direction. This allows the sleep physician or service provider to change pressure or other settings in the PAP machine remotely. In some countries, this is not legal, but in other countries, where long distance bridging is a challenge (eg, Australia), this currently is in practice.

Diagnostic tools, such as data transmission, and the use of home sleep apnea testing and use of wearables and sleep apps are a broad field of telemedicine application within sleep medicine. They are discussed previously. For these applications, telemedicine is an integrated and embedded tool that nobody ever worries about or even denotes as telemedicine. This tool generally is accepted.

Final and relatively new aspects of telemedicine with sleep medicine, which have become used more frequently during the recent pandemic, are teleconsulting and video counseling with patients. Usually the physician-patient relationship in sleep medicine is personal, and the medical interview and sleep test results discussion are very personal. The pandemic made it necessary, however, to introduce distant medical interviews with and without video support. Questionnaires were applied as usual and help in assessing the symptoms and complaints. All data collected then are saved in electronic health care records. For these records, the recently amended General Data Protection Regulation needs to be considered. The electronic health care record structure is consolidated in Europe according to new recommendations regarding the structure as developed by

European Committee for Standardization. Plans are developed to create a cloud for health care records, which are accessible with a 2-key encryption by a physician or health care provider and the patient. This kind of data storage is developed for sleep medicine as well, with consideration for storing recorded sleep data, not just report data. The extensive usage of digital solutions in the field of sleep medicine makes this interdisciplinary specialty devoted to chronic disorders a first-line field for an integrated health care records, including consolidated reports and signals.

SUMMARY

Sleep is without doubt an important interdisciplinary field of medicine. Some disorders have a high prevalence and pose a burden on global health care. Outstanding in this regard is sleep apnea.[34] Other sleep disorders like insomnia, with a similarly high prevalence, may require less device-driven diagnostic tools.

Different fields of biomedical engineering and medical informatics have come together and can help advance the interdisciplinary field of sleep medicine. The challenges are in components of hardware and software. The technical developments made in electronics and in computational methodologies and computational power can be used and exploited to move sleep medicine forward in terms of better understanding of sleep per se and in better service for patient care.

CLINICS CARE POINTS

- Currently, visual sleep staging remains state of the art. New algorithms, however, based on probability, in the near future will be able to support visual sleep staging.

- Sensor developments in devices used for home sleep testing have taken large steps recently in delivering information for health risks and phenotyping of patients.

- Sensor developments linked to wearables and smartphones have inaugurated a more convenient, contact-free sleep recording that is accessible anywhere and at low cost—clinical use remains unclear.

- Telemedicine in sleep medicine can be used to bridge long distances and improve patient management strategies but cannot replace the intimate patient/physician relationship in exploring health problems.

DISCLOSURE

T. Penzel received funding for research by Cidelec, Löwenstein Medical. He received speaker fees from Löwenstein Medical, Neuwirth Medical, and Jazz Pharma. He is an advisory board member of Bayer Pharma, Cerebra, Nukute, and Jazz Pharma. He holds shares from Advanced Sleep Research, Nukute, and The Siestagroup GmbH. This research was funded partially by a grant by Löwenstein Foundation. This work was supported by the European Commission's H2020 research and innovation programme Project No. 826093 (ASCLEPIOS).

REFERENCES

1. Rechtschaffen A, Kales AA. Manual of standardized terminology, techniques, and scoring system for sleep stages of human subjects. Bethesda: US Department of Health, Education, and Welfare Public Health Service – National Institute of Health; 1968.
2. Danker-Hopfe H, Gruber G, Kunz D, et al. Interrater reliability between scorers from eight European sleep laboratories in subjects with different sleep disorders. J Sleep Res 2004;13:63–9.
3. Penzel T, Hirshkowitz M, Harsh J, et al. Digital analysis and technical specifications. J Clin Sleep Med 2007;3:109–20.
4. Berry RB, Quan SF, Abreu AR, et al. for the American Academy of sleep medicine: the AASM manual for the scoring of sleep and associated events: rules, terminology and technical specifications. Version 2.6. Darien: American Academy of Sleep Medicine; 2020.
5. Anderer P, Gruber G, Parapatics S, et al. An E-health solution for automatic sleep classification according to rechtschaffen and Kales: validation study of the somnolyzer 24 x 7 utilizing the siesta database. Neuropsychobiology 2005;51:115–33.
6. Younes M, Ostrowski M, Soiferman M, et al. Odds ratio product of sleep EEG as a continuous measure of sleep state. Sleep 2015;38(4):641–54.
7. Lim DC, Mazzotti DR, Sutherland K, et al. Reinventing polysomnography in the age of precision medicine. Sleep Med Rev 2020;52:101313.
8. Mazzotti DR, Lim DC, Sutherland K, et al. Opportunities for utilizing polysomnography signals to characterize obstructive sleep apnea subtypes and severity. Physiol Meas 2018;39:09TR01.
9. Stephansen JB, Olesen AN, Olsen M, et al. Neural network analysis of sleep stages enables efficient diagnosis of narcolepsy. Nat Commun 2018;9:5229.
10. Penzel T, Malberg H. Technologische entwicklungen in der Schlafmedizin. Somnologie 2017;21:91–2.
11. Salmi T, Telakivi T, Partinen M. Evaluation of automatic analysis of SCSB, airflow, and oxygen

saturation signals in patients with sleep related apneas. Chest 1989;96:255–61.

12. Paalasmaa J, Toivonen H, Partinen M. Adaptive heartbeat modeling for beat-to-beat heart rate measurement in ballistocardiograms. IEEE J Biomed Health Inform 2015;19:1945–52.

13. De Chazal P, Fox N, O'Hare E. Sleep/wake measurement using a non-contact biomotion sensor. J Sleep Res 2011;20:356–66.

14. Gehring J, Gesche H, Drewniok G, et al. Nocturnal blood pressure fluctuations measured by using pulse transit time in patients with severe obstructive sleep apnea syndrome. Sleep Breath 2018;22:337–43.

15. Sommermeyer D, Zou D, Ficker JH, et al. Detection of cardiovascular risk from a photoplethysmographic signal using a matching pursuit algorithm. Med Biol Eng Comput 2016;54:1111–21.

16. Schnall RP, Shlitner A, Sheffy J, et al. Periodic profound peripheral vasoconstriction – a new marker of obstructive sleep apnea. Sleep 1999;22:939–46.

17. Lavie P, Schnall RP, Sheffy J, et al. Peripheral vasoconstriction during REM sleep detected by a new plethysmographic method. Nat Med 2000;6:606.

18. Yalamanchali S, Farajian V, Hamilton C, et al. Diagnosis of obstructive sleep apnea by peripheral arterial tonometry meta-analysis. JAMA Otolaryngol Head Neck Surg 2013;139(12):1343–50.

19. Pillar G, Berall M, Berry R, et al. Detecting central sleep apnea in adult patients using watch-PAT – a multicenter validation study. Sleep Breath 2019. https://doi.org/10.1007/s11325-019-01904-5.

20. Glos M, Sabil A, Jelavic KS, et al. Characterization of respiratory events in obstructive sleep apnea using suprasternal pressure monitoring. J Clin Sleep Med 2018;14:359–69.

21. Sabil A, Schöbel C, Glos M, et al. Apnea and hypopnea characterization using esophageal pressure, respiratory inductance plethysmography, and suprasternal pressure: a comparative study. Sleep and Breathing 2019;23:1169–76.

22. Fietze I, Penzel T, Alonderis A, et al. Management of obstructive sleep apnea in Europe. Sleep Med 2011; 12:190–7.

23. Verbraecken J, Hedner J, Penzel T. Pre-operative screening for obstructive sleep apnoea. Eur Respir Rev 2017;26:160012.

24. American Sleep Disorders Association (ASDA). Practice Parameters for the use of portable recording in the assessment of obstructive sleep apnea. Sleep 1994;17:372–7.

25. Collop NA, Tracy SL, Kapur V, et al. Obstructive sleep apnea devices for out-of-center (OOC) testing: technology evaluation. J Clin Sleep Med 2011;7:531–48.

26. Sadeh A, Alster J, Urbach D, et al. Actigraphically based automatic bedtime sleep-wake scoring: validity and clinical applications. J Amb Monit 1989;2: 209–16.

27. Gu W, Shangguan L, Yang Z, et al. Sleep hunter: towards fine grained sleep stage tracking with smartphones. IEEE Trans mobile Comput 2016;15(6): 1514–27.

28. Penzel T, Fietze I, Glos M. Alternative algorithms and devices in sleep apnoea diagnosis: what we know and what we expect. Curr Opin Pulm Med 2020; 26:650–6.

29. Khosla S, Deak MC, Gault D, et al, American Academy of Sleep Medicine Board of Directors. Consumer sleep technology: an American Academy of Sleep Medicine position statement. J Clin Sleep Med 2018;14(5):877–80.

30. Elison S, Ward J, Williams C, et al. Feasibility of a UK community-based, eTherapy mental health service in greater manchester: repeated measures and between-groups study of 'living life to the full interactive', 'sleepio' and 'breaking free online' at 'self help services'. BMJ Open 2017;7:e016392.

31. Woehrle H, Ficker JH, Graml A, et al. Telemedicine-based proactive patient management during positive airway pressure therapy Impact on therapy termination rate. Adherence monitoring. Somnologie 2017;21:121–7.

32. Hirshkowitz M. Polysomnography challenges. Sleep Med Clin 2016;11:403–11.

33. Penzel T, Schöbel C, Fietze I. New technology to assess sleep apnea: wearables, smartphones, and accessories. F1000Res 2018;7:413.

34. Benjafield AV, Ayas NT, Eastwood PR, et al. Estimating the global prevalence and burden of obstructive sleep apnoea: a literature-based analysis. Lancet Respir Med 2019;7:687–98.

Sleep and Cardiovascular Risk

Lyudmila Korostovtseva, MD, PhD[a],*, Mikhail Bochkarev, MD, PhD[b], Yurii Sviryaev, MD, PhD[c]

KEYWORDS

- Sleep health • Sleep disorders • Sleep timing • Cardiovascular health • Cardiovascular risk
- Cardiovascular prevention • Cardiometabolic diseases

KEY POINTS

- Sleep is essential for healthy being and healthy functioning of human body.
- Sleep is a multidimensional concept.
- Sleep disorders and sleep deprivation are associated with the deterioration in human body functioning and increased cardiovascular risks.
- Cardiovascular functioning depends on multidimensional characteristics of sleep.

INTRODUCTION

The recent guidelines for cardiovascular prevention released by the American College of Cardiology/American Heart Association (2019) state that counseling on sleep and sleep hygiene (along with an advice on physical activity) should be provided to prevent cardiovascular diseases (CVD).[1] Thus, sleep hygiene should be addressed within prevention and/or treatment approaches in obesity, whereas sleep duration and sleep quality should be considered as potential therapeutic targets in subjects with high blood pressure (BP). Interestingly, guidelines of the European Society of Cardiology (2016) on cardiovascular prevention do not consider sleep per se (but obstructive sleep apnea only) as a target for preventive measures.[2]

The recent data evidence a relationship between sleep and CVD, with the focus on the association between sleep disorders and cardiovascular pathology. Thus, despite the controversial results of the interventional trials, there is no doubt that obstructive sleep apnea (OSA) is a predictor of CVD or their progression,

including hypertension, cardiac arrhythmias, and atherosclerotic heart disease.[3–5] Insomnia and sleep deprivation are also related to increased cardiometabolic risks.[6] Both short and long sleep were shown to be associated with the unfavorable outcomes.[6–8]

Accumulating evidence suggests that healthy sleep is not only the absence of evident sleep disorders or sleep-related complaints. Sleep is a heterogeneous and a highly structured state. In 2014, Buysse[9] suggested to distinguish 5 dimensions to characterize sleep health: satisfaction, alertness, timing, efficiency, and duration. The concept of sleep health includes a broader spectrum of multidimensional features and considers not only sleep duration, sleep stages, and phases but also such characteristics as microstructure of sleep, sleep timing, sleep efficiency, self-perception of sleep, napping, and others.[10,11] Matricciani and colleagues[10] distinguished 4 sleep profiles based on complex analysis of actigraphy data: short sleepers, late to bed, long sleepers, and overall good sleepers. Compared with the last one, the first 3 profiles seemed to be associated with less

[a] Sleep Laboratory, Research Department for Hypertension, Department for Cardiology, Almazov National Medical Research Centre, 2 Akkuratov Street, St Petersburg 197341, Russia; [b] Sleep Laboratory, Research Department for Hypertension, Almazov National Medical Research Centre, 2 Akkuratov Street, St Petersburg 197341, Russia; [c] Research Department for Hypertension, Almazov National Medical Research Centre, 2 Akkuratov Street, St Petersburg 197341, Russia
* Corresponding author.
E-mail address: korostovtseva_ls@almazovcentre.ru

Sleep Med Clin 16 (2021) 485–497
https://doi.org/10.1016/j.jsmc.2021.05.001
1556-407X/21/© 2021 Elsevier Inc. All rights reserved.

favorable cardiometabolic health. The markers included BP, body mass index, apolipoproteins, glycoprotein acetyls, and composite metabolic syndrome severity score. Montag and colleagues[12] in the Chicago Area Sleep Study showed that increased risk for hypertension had a tighter association with the objective and subjective sleep quality estimates rather than objective actigraphy-based sleep duration. Sleep timing was found to be predictive for weight status[13,14] and insulin resistance,[15] which might be mediated by dietary intake,[16] whereas lower sleep regularity is associated with the higher risks of diabetes mellitus.[17] Cardiovascular risks related to napping provoked discussion due to controversial results.[18–22] Self-reported poor quality of sleep is related to higher risks of hypertension, coronary artery disease,[23] and diabetes mellitus, whereas good restfulness from sleep is associated with lower risks of CVD (eg, stroke, myocardial infarction, angina pectoris, heart failure, atrial fibrillation).[24]

Therefore, we can assume that the lowest cardiovascular risks would apply to subjects with normal sleep assessed by multimodal approach. However, even healthy subjects might manifest some sleep-related cardiovascular risks.

CARDIOVASCULAR REGULATION AND RISKS IN NORMAL SLEEP
Cardiovascular Oscillations in Normal Sleep

In normal sleep, higher risks are attributed to rapid eye movement (REM) sleep, which is characterized by the abrupt surges in heart rate (HR) and BP (up to the levels in wakefulness and higher) and increased variability of these parameters (**Table 1**).[25,26] REM sleep is also accompanied by the increase in peripheral tone (eg, vasoconstriction of the arterioles in the fingers).[27]

On the contrary, non-REM (NREM) sleep (or slow wave sleep [SWS]) is associated with the decrease in BP, HR, cardiac output, and systemic vascular resistance, and, as a consequence, vasodilation, which also contributes to BP drop. These effects mainly mediate the normal HR and BP reduction during sleep (although circadian effects play an important role as well in the formation of the "dipping" BP pattern), which achieves 10% to 20% reduction compared with wakefulness in healthy individuals. Moreover, the lack of SWS (eg, due to sleep apnea and other sleep disorders) was shown to be associated with higher risk of cardiovascular dysfunction, especially increased risk of hypertension.[28]

The changes in coronary and cerebral blood flow are also different in REM and NREM sleep.

Some experimental studies suggest a decrease in visceral blood flow from wakefulness to NREM sleep (because of a reduced metabolic demand) and its increase in REM sleep (in particular, in phasic episodes, as a response to increased metabolism and visceral functional activation),[29–32] whereas other studies describe opposite changes.[33] However, most researchers agree that REM sleep is characterized by higher variability and abrupt fluctuations of cardiovascular indices, which can result in higher cardiovascular risks.[33,34] The opposite cardiovascular and metabolic effects in NREM and REM sleep support the hypothesis of reallocation of energy for different physiologic needs and processes during different sleep stages and wakefulness.[35,36]

The fluctuations in cardiovascular functioning are mediated by various mechanisms that interact with each other, including autonomic changes, central neural circuits, circadian variations, changes in endocrine activity, and other mechanisms.[30]

Regulation of Cardiovascular Functions in Normal Sleep

Autonomic nervous system plays a major role in the regulation of cardiovascular functions during sleep. NREM sleep is characterized by the predominant vagal activity, increased baroreceptor gain and relative stability of autonomic regulation, as well as the decrease in sympathetic activity downgrading from stage N1 to N3.[37–41] As a result, the onset of NREM sleep is accompanied by the aforementioned vasodilation and gradual decrease in HR and BP. In healthy individuals, normal sinus arrhythmia and cardiorespiratory coupling are registered. REM sleep is also associated with predominantly parasympathetic activation; however, during phasic episodes, abrupt and profound sympathetic surges, low baroreceptor gain, and suppression of cardiac efferent vagal tone are registered.[39,42] As a result, REM-related sudden fluctuations in HR are followed by its deceleration mediated through baroreflex mechanism. These episodes manifest as sinus arrhythmia and alternating episodes of bradycardia and intermittent tachycardia. On the other hand, during tonic phase of REM sleep abrupt decelerations in HR are observed independently from respiratory changes; they are abolished by the muscarinic blockade suggesting their vagal-related genesis.

The BP increases in REM sleep partly result from the sympathetic-driven vasoconstriction in skeletal muscles, which is opposed by vasodilation in the mesenteric and renal vasculature. Moreover, short central apneas, obstructive apneas, and

Table 1
Cardiovascular regulation in normal sleep

Parameter	Non-REM Sleep	REM Sleep
Heart rate	Reduction Cyclical respiratory-related variations	Abrupt surges Increased variability
Blood pressure	Reduction Cyclical respiratory-related variations	Abrupt surges Increased variability
Cardiac output	Reduction	Increase
Systemic vascular resistance	Reduction (vasodilation)	Increase (vasoconstriction)
Renal and mesenteric vascular conductance	Increase	Variable (more vasodilation)
Cerebral blood flow	Depends on the region	Depends on the region (more vasodilation)
Coronary blood flow	Reduction	Abrupt increases

hypopneas are common during phasic REM sleep, which, in turn, can enhance HR and BP changes.[39,42–44]

Episodic fluctuations in coronary blood flow registered during REM sleep are presumably associated with the HR increase and decrease in coronary vascular resistance; they are mediated by the increased alpha-adrenergic discharge and are independent of respiration and other factors.[43,45]

Central nervous system, including cortical and medullar neural networks, is involved in the regulation of sleep onset and the switch between sleep stages, as well as in cardiovascular regulation. Importantly, central regulation of autonomic balance seems to be independent of peripheral sympathetic innervation as shown in studies with partial and complete spinal cord lesions.[46–48] The hypothalamus plays a key role, with sleep-promoting neurons located in its preoptic region and wake-promoting neurons found in the posterior hypothalamus.[49] Among brain structures involved both in sleep regulation and in cardiovascular control the most important are serotoninergic neurons of the midline raphe of the pons, the orbital frontal cortex, hippocampus, hypothalamus, and amygdala. Insular cortex regulates cardiovascular functions in both sleep and wakefulness through modulation of sympathetic and parasympathetic activity. Cerebellum regulates BP through vestibular/cerebellar ways providing BP maintenance in postural changes. Central autonomic mechanisms (central nervous system excitation) play important role in abrupt HR and BP fluctuations during REM sleep.[41,50] Moreover, the suprachiasmatic nucleus (SCN) of the hypothalamus is the main pacemaker for the circadian rhythms, as well as of all cardiometabolic processes. Via vasopressin, produced by the neurons of the supraoptic and paraventricular nuclei, the hypothalamus regulates fluid and electrolyte homeostasis, circulating blood volume, and BP.

In sleep, arousals (rapid transient episodes of cortical activation and/or autonomic activation, which are either spontaneous or a reaction to the external stimuli), lead to brief transient surges in sympathetic activity, vascular tone, BP, and HR usually followed by their decrease.[51,52] Similarly, large body movements, dreaming, and auditory stimuli (present in healthy sleepers) not leading to the evident cortical arousal can exert autonomic reactions. Similar responses are found in relation to ultradian variations in sleep electroencephalography (EEG) (ie, arousals, K-complexes, delta wave bursts), which supports the direct role of central autonomic drive to the heart and vascular beds.

Reflexogenous regulation includes cardiorespiratory, baroreceptor, and chemoreceptor coupling. Cardiorespiratory coupling mediates peripheral vasodilation and decreased sympathetic renal stimulation, as well as fluctuations in the circulating blood volume and BP in response to postural changes and fluid shift.[53] Baroreflex (baroreceptors in the carotid bodies and aortic arch) mediates rapid cardiovascular response to the BP-related aortic and carotid stretch via sympathoinhibitory and direct cardioinhibitory effects.[25,26,41] Chemoreflexes are activated by changes in blood gases: hypercapnia stimulates central chemoreceptors (in the medulla oblongata), whereas both hypoxia and hypercapnia activate peripheral chemoreceptors (in the carotid bodies). Consequently, sympathetic nerve drive is induced, leading to BP elevation and stimulating respiratory center causing hyperventilation. Peripheral chemoreflex can also increase vagal tone resulting in bradycardia. Hypoxic and hypercapnic responses depend on the vigilance-sleep state, being maximal in wakefulness, intermediate in NREM sleep, and minimal in REM sleep. In addition, chemoreceptor regulation plays an important role in the modulation of cerebral blood flow in response to carbon dioxide fluctuations and might be involved in the development of cerebrovascular pathologic condition.[54]

Endocrine regulation of sleep and cardiovascular system includes the growth hormone axis, the corticotropic axis, the thyroid axis, prolactin, and the gonadal axis, as well as leptin and ghrelin. All these components are also involved in the glucose and lipid metabolism closely related to cardiovascular health. These components demonstrate clear day-night and/or sleep-wakefulness patterns.[55] SWS (predominantly, the first half of night in healthy subjects) is associated with anabolic effects and energy saving, increased lipid and fatty acids mobilization, gluconeogenesis in liver, decreased tissue glucose uptake, and increased insulin secretion, whereas the second half of the night is characterized by the higher activity of contrainsular hormones.[49,53,56–59] Melatonin, hormone secreted by the pineal gland, is known to regulate BP and vascular tone and might be involved in nocturnal BP drop.[60,61] Moreover, melatonin exerts cardioprotective action through antioxidant, antiinflammatory, antiatherogenic, and hypolipidemic effects. Being a key regulator of inner clocks it is involved in the circadian variations of cardiometabolic parameters, and the impairment in melatonin release might be associated with higher cardiovascular risks.[60,61] With regard to the renin-angiotensin-aldosterone system, which is a major participant in BP regulation, the decreases in plasma renin activity are synchronized with the REM sleep, and the enhanced activity is associated with SWS in healthy individuals. Via interrelation with autonomic nervous system it mediates volume-dependent mechanisms of BP regulation.[49,53,62]

Circadian regulation includes a central pacemaker in the brain (SCN entrained by light), which directly controls and synchronizes the activity of different components of the cardiovascular system,[63] and several clocks in peripheral tissues, which integrate signals from the central pacemaker and external (light, physical activity, food intake, etc.) and endogenous stimuli and regulate visceral functions and hormonal secretion. Clock genes (eg, the CLOCK gene—circadian locomotor output cycles kaput gene, BMAL1, Per, and Cry) play an important role in the modulation of cardiovascular functioning and metabolism.[64–67] These genes are modulated by endocrine stimuli, in particular, via the hypothalamic-pituitary-adrenal axis and melatonin.[68] However, light might influence BP independently of melatonin secretion.[69,70] Moreover, the association between cardiometabolic functions and circadian rhythms is bidirectional. Therefore, feeding time, diet, physical activity, and energy expenditure may shift gene expression followed by the modification of cardiometabolic processes.[71] It should be noted that diurnal fluctuations in various biologic parameters, including vascular tone, catecholamine secretion, BP, HR, and blood coagulability factors, are present independently of any other factors, which was proved in desynchrony protocol studies,[37,38,66,72] and might be potential triggers for cardiovascular accidents.[73]

Cardiovascular Physiologic Sleep-Related Responses and Risks

Sometimes the physiologic sleep-related responses might have deleterious effects. Resulting from the imbalance in autonomic control and abrupt increases in vagal tone occurring in REM sleep,[44] healthy individuals may demonstrate severe bradycardia (<40 bpm) in up to 24%, first- and second-degree atrioventricular (AV) block (>10%), and sinus pauses (<2–2.5 seconds, 4%–10%) associated with REM sleep and/or NREM-REM shifts.[44,74,75] These bradyarrhythmias are considered benign and are common in young subjects, professional athletes, and people doing rough labor. In general, they do not require interventions but monitoring. However, one should consider conditions predisposing to higher risk of threatening arrhythmias in subjects with sleep-related bradyarrhythmias, in particular, due to triggered activity provoked by abrupt sympathetic surges. Thus underlying (and in many cases underdiagnosed) structural heart damage, some medications (eg, antiarrhythmic drugs III class), endothelial dysfunction, cardiac ion channel disorders,[76] and (latent) long QT (LQT) syndrome (type 3 LQT syndrome)[77] can lead to nocturnal threatening cardiac arrhythmic events (eg, torsades de pointes) and sudden cardiac death in subjects with otherwise benign sleep-related bradyarrhythmias.[4,78] Pathologic sleep-related bradyarrhythmias include severe bradycardia less than 20 to 30 bpm, sinus pauses greater than 3 seconds, AV block II degree Mobitz 2, and AV block III degree. Koehler and colleagues[79] confirmed an uneven distribution of severe, clinically significant bradyarrhythmias (AV block III, sinus arrest) during sleep with their predominance in REM sleep compared with NREM sleep.[80] In subjects with autonomic dysfunction and vagal predominance, these mechanisms can underlie the development of severe REM-related bradyarrhythmias, including long asystoles. In most cases, electrophysiological studies demonstrate normal sinus node function and atrioventricular conduction.[44] However, bradyarrhythmias can be exacerbated in patients with concomitant pathologic conditions, including coronary heart disease and OSA,[81] which should be considered when approaching a patient with nocturnal heart rhythm disturbances. An individualized approach is required; anticholinergic drugs and implantable pacemakers are considered treatment options.

Profound BP drop in NREM sleep and "overdipping" BP pattern due to the vagal activation might be deleterious for patients with severe coronary heart disease and cerebral atherosclerosis leading to myocardial or cerebral ischemia, especially in the presence of endothelial dysfunction. On the other hand, vagal-related bradycardia and improved myocardial perfusion might be protective, but this needs to be proven.[82] Loss of physiologic BP decrease at night (nondipping profile) is also associated with higher rates of cardiovascular morbidity and mortality,[83,84] and the approaches aimed at normalization of circadian BP profile have been largely investigated.

Chemoreflex and baroreflex response can be altered in comorbid pathologies, such as sleep apnea, cardiometabolic diseases (heart failure, obesity[85]), and aortic diseases (carotid atherosclerosis, carotid endovascular interventions, such as endarterectomy and stenting[85,86]) resulting in sympathetic overdrive and reduced vasoreactivity.[87–89] The carotid body denervation, suggested as a treatment approach in sympathetic-related pathologic conditions (heart failure, resistant hypertension, OSA, etc.[90]), does not lead to the development of respiratory disturbances when unilateral intervention is performed, which might be explained by the chemoreflex plasticity in the remnant carotid artery. However, bilateral removal of carotid bodies increases susceptibility to irregular breathing, in particular in sleep, which might increase cardiovascular risks.[91]

The diurnal (24-hour) distribution of acute cardiovascular events is uneven, with the clear peaks observed at early morning and early evening hours. The double-peak 24-hour pattern is observed for most acute cardiovascular accidents, including sudden cardiac death, cardiac arrhythmias,[92,93] myocardial infarction,[94] stroke,[95] pulmonary embolism,[96] acute aortic dissections,[97] and others, although specific timing can vary between the certain pathologic conditions.[98,99] Thus, among inpatients the highest rates of cardiac arrest are registered between 02:00 and 03:00 AM (odds ratio [OR] 3.06) and 06:00 and 07:00 AM (OR 1.95),

whereas the lowest level is between 20:00 and 21:00 PM (OR 0.42).[100] In the retrospective study by Ramireddy and colleagues,[101] 22.3% of all sudden cardiac deaths (n = 4126) in the general population occurred at nighttime. The time preference in the occurrence of most cardiovascular events is mainly independent of demographic characteristics, comorbidities, and potential pathophysiological causes.[99] However, Ramireddy and colleagues[101] found that nighttime deaths compared with the daytime cases were characterized by lower rates of restoration of spontaneous circulation and lower survival rate; female sex, intake of medications affecting central nervous system, and concomitant chronic obstructive pulmonary disease/asthma appeared to be the independent predictors of nocturnal sudden cardiac death in the multivariate analysis.[102]

The unfavorable outcomes of nocturnal events can be explained by the lower availability of health care services and surveillance levels and other environmental triggers. These outcomes can also be attributed to sleep disorders, primarily OSA and nocturnal hypoxemia causing myocardial or cerebral ischemia[103,104]; the pharmacokinetics and pharmacodynamics of the medications; and other factors.[105] At the same time the blunted or imbalanced 24-hour patterns in physiologic processes (variations in hormone secretion, vascular tone, HR, BP, coagulability, inflammatory activity, and others) should be considered as a major cause of the diurnal patterns of cardiovascular events. Thus, higher morning BP surges and absence of nocturnal BP dip are the well-known predictors of cardiovascular events.[106,107] Similarly, a blunted decrease in nocturnal HR predicts the risk of all-cause mortality and fatal and nonfatal cardiovascular events.[108] Prothrombotic factors, including powerful inhibitor of fibrinolysis plasminogen activator inhibitor-1 (PAI-1), show clear 24-hour rhythmicity with the early morning peak at about 06:30 AM increasing the risk of thrombotic events in susceptible subjects.[109,110] This observation is also true for some anticoagulation factors (tissue factor pathway inhibitor[111]), suggesting that an impaired balance between prothrombotic and antithrombotic molecules, as well as the interference of other factors (eg, sleep disorders, including mild sleep impairment[112]) might play a key role in cardiovascular accidents.

CARDIOVASCULAR RISKS IN SLEEP DISORDERS

The available evidence on the main CVDs associated with the common sleep disorders is summarized in **Table 2**.

Table 2
Sleep disorders and cardiovascular risks

Sleep Disorder	Association	Reference
Sleep-disordered breathing	Hypertension Cardiac arrhythmias Metabolic consequences (diabetes mellitus) (?)	3,5,6,74
Insomnia	Autonomic dysregulation Hypertension	113–115
Sleep deprivation and sleep fragmentation	Hypertension (?) Metabolic consequences (diabetes mellitus) (?)	1,6
Periodic limb movements	Autonomic activation BP surges Increased cardiovascular risk (controversial data)	116,117
Parasomnias	No conclusive data Potential relation between nocturnal eating syndrome and metabolic disorders and obesity	118,119
REM-sleep behavior disorder	Lack of data Association with the risk of stroke (a large Korean population)	119
Narcolepsy, hypersomnias	Impairment of autonomic regulation, high risk of obesity and metabolic disorders	7,120–122
Circadian misalignment	Cardiometabolic changes, increased risk of diabetes mellitus	113,123–125

Question marks denote the available evidence is controversial and/ or very limited.

CARDIOVASCULAR HEALTH AS A FUNCTION OF SLEEP

Among various functions of sleep (cognitive performance, memory consolidation, metabolism regulation, immune function, emotional processing, dreaming, regulation of pain, and others), the maintenance of cardiovascular health is not usually taken into account.[126] Is it a separate function or does it result from other processes occurring during sleep?

A potential clue is provided by the visceral theory of sleep and the theory of clearance and restorative function of sleep, carried out via the glymphatic system.

The visceral theory of sleep considers that all sensory brain areas that process the signals coming from the environment and motor activity (somatosensory, visual, auditory signals and others) in wakefulness, in sleep switch to the processing of internal signals coming from the visceral organs (interoceptive stimuli). The aim of this processing is visceral

diagnostics and functional restoration.[50,127–131] The theory implies that various interoceptive (visceral) stimuli can evoke changes in brain activity manifesting in EEG oscillations.[127,128,132]

This hypothesis was confirmed by a series of animal experiments involving visceral electrostimulation and registration of visceral spontaneous activity. Although most experiments demonstrated the association of brain sleep activity and gastrointestinal tract signals, there are few studies that consider the link between cardiovascular system signals and cortical activity. Thus Lavrova and colleagues[129] observed typical cortical response related to R wave on the electrocardiography (ECG) in sleeping cats with the latent period 40 to 120 milliseconds. Intriguingly, these cortical responses were observed only in SWS and never when the animals were awake.

These findings are supported by human studies that demonstrated a coupling between slow EEG oscillations and heartbeat and arterial pulsation signal of near-infrared spectroscopy.[128] This coupling is the most evident during sleep. Similar findings were demonstrated by Lechinger and colleagues[133] and Forouzanfar and colleagues[134] who interpreted them as the interaction between central and autonomic nervous system coupled with respiration and systolic BP. However, the investigators cannot assert whether the EEG oscillations are modulated by cardiac-induced oscillations or modulate HR. Brindle and colleagues[135] based on the clinical data came to a conclusion that SWS can modulate cardiovascular stress reactivity and ameliorate deleterious daytime stress-related effects.

These experiments and clinical observations confirm the hypothesis about association between visceral systems functioning and sensory information processing during sleep; however, we still do not know how this association and the processing change in CVD and whether there is association between primary cardiovascular pathology and sleep disruption (in particular, SWS disruption), or vice versa (whether primary sleep disorder leads to cardiovascular abnormal functioning). Thus Kwon and colleagues[136] showed that patients with atrial fibrillation have lower slow wave activity; however, it is not clear which changes—CVD or blunted sleep—are primary and which ones are secondary.

The discovery of *the glymphatic system* and its role in waste clearance of brain during sleep, mainly during SWS, provoked a burst of studies investigating the relation between disordered sleep and glymphatic function, with the primary focus on neurodegenerative diseases.[137,138] However, we can speculate that it may be also involved in the regulation of cardiovascular and cerebrovascular functions, thus taking part in the maintenance of cardiovascular health or exerting cardiovascular risks in case of the clearance system damage. Experimental studies demonstrated a negative correlation between glymphatic influx and HR. This correlation can be simply explained by the changes in cardiovascular functioning during SWS, because there was a positive correlation with EEG delta power.[139] Nevertheless, an independent association with cardiovascular regulation might also matter. A potential mechanism can involve the system of apolipoprotein E (APOE) and APOE gene variants, which are known to be associated with cardiometabolic disorders, for example, dyslipidemia and insulin resistance,[140–142] and water-permeable channels aquaporins,[143] including aquaporin 4, which is a key participant controlling bidirectional fluid exchange between the blood-brain barrier and blood-cerebrospinal fluid barrier.[143]

INTERVENTIONS TO DECREASE SLEEP-RELATED CARDIOVASCULAR RISKS

We still lack understanding whether any medication or nonmedication approaches for sleep improvement and modulation would allow for CVD prevention and treatment. Nevertheless, healthy sleep hygiene and appropriate sleep duration should be recommended for both primary cardiovascular prevention in the general population and secondary prevention.[1,6,144,145]

Chronotherapeutical approaches were shown to be effective. In particular, specific timing of certain medications with regard to the circadian variations of physiologic parameters and pharmacokinetic and pharmacodynamic features of the drugs leads to their higher efficiency. However, the current data are mainly focused on short-term effects on BP,[146,147] whereas the evidence on the long-term prognostic impact of such approaches is rather scarce.[148]

Dietary melatonin supplementation is associated with favorable cardiometabolic changes, including improved lipid profile[149,150] and glucose metabolism.[151] Experimental studies show that melatonin can ameliorate insulin resistance and reverse cardiovascular remodeling.[152,153] Owing to its potent antihypertensive effect, melatonin is recommended as a dietary supplement in subjects with nocturnal hypertension.[150]

Nonmedication interventions, in particular, physical exercise, are known to affect sleep and the diurnal fluctuations of biologically active molecules. Regarding physical exercise the response might be dependent not on the maximal duration of the exercise and exertion, but rather on the relative intensity compared with the subject's maximal exercise capacity and exercise timing.[154] The recent findings suggest that other approaches such as light therapy[155,156] and shift in feeding schedule can affect both sleep and physiologic processes,[111] including coagulation factors secretion, glucose metabolism,[156] and BP. Neurostimulation techniques (transcranial electrical and magnetic stimulation; acoustic stimulation, including music listening; etc.) can help to enhance sleep and, in particular, SWS.[157,158] Moreover, such interventions are associated with the change in autonomic activity with increase in parasympathetic tone and a change in cortisol levels,[159] which might have cardiometabolic effects. Some experimental techniques, for example, adenosine A2A receptor agonists are also promising.[160] Despite promising results, the effects of these interventions on cardiovascular risks and long-term prognosis are not clear and need further investigation.

SUMMARY

In conclusion, sleep is essential for healthy being and healthy functioning of the human body as a whole, as well as of each organ and system. Sleep disorders, such as sleep-disordered breathing, insomnia, sleep fragmentation, and sleep deprivation are associated with the deterioration in human body functioning and increased cardiovascular risks. However, owing to the complex regulation and heterogeneous state sleep per se can be associated with cardiovascular dysfunction in susceptible subjects. The understanding of sleep as a multidimensional concept is important for better prevention and treatment of CVD.

CLINICS CARE POINTS

- When evaluating results of 24-hour ECG monitoring, pay attention to the night/day (and sleep/wakefulness) ratio of heart rhythm disorders. In most cases, these arrhythmias are benign. However, consider conditions predisposing to higher risk of threatening heart rhythm disorders (eg, structural heart damage, some medications, endothelial dysfunction, cardiac ion channel disorders, and long QT syndrome including latent forms).
- When evaluating 24-hour ambulatory blood pressure monitoring, pay attention to the circadian blood pressure profile. Excessive blood pressure drop at night (overdipping pattern), which is considered generally normal, might be deleterious in subjects with coronary heart disease and cerebral atherosclerosis.
- In clinical routine, when prescribing medications and other treatment interventions, consider 24-h pattern in physiologic parameters and processes (variations in heart rate, blood pressure, hormone secretion, vascular tone, coagulability, inflammatory activity, etc.).

DISCLOSURE

The authors have nothing to disclose.

FUNDING

This work is supported by the Ministry of Science and Higher Education of the Russian Federation (Agreement No. 075-15-2020-901).

REFERENCES

1. 2019 ACC/AHA guideline on the primary prevention of cardiovascular disease. *J Am* Coll Cardiol 2019;74(10):e177–231.
2. 2016 European Guidelines on cardiovascular disease prevention in clinical practice. Eur Heart J 2016;37(29):2315–81.
3. Agabiti E, France MA, Uk AD, et al. 2018 ESC/ESH Guidelines for the management of arterial hypertension the Task Force for the management of arterial hypertension of the European Society of Cardiology (ESC) and the European Society of. Eur Heart J 2018;39:3021–104.
4. 2013 ESC Guidelines on cardiac pacing and cardiac resynchronization therapy the Task Force on cardiac pacing and resynchronization therapy of the. Eur Heart J 2013;34:2281–329.
5. 2020 ESC Guidelines for the diagnosis and management of atrial fibrillation developed in collaboration with the European Association of Cardio-Thoracic Surgery (EACTS) the Task Force for the diagnosis and management of atrial fibrillation of the Europea. Eur Heart J 2020;1–126.
6. American diabetes association standards of medical care in diabetes - 2019. Diabetes Care 2019; 42(Suppl):S1–193.
7. Beaman A, Bhide MC, Mchill AW, et al. Biological pathways underlying the association between habitual long-sleep and elevated cardiovascular risk in adults. Sleep Med 2021;78:135–40.
8. Butler MJ, Spruill TM, Johnson DA, et al. Suboptimal sleep and incident cardiovascular disease among African Americans in the Jackson Heart Study (JHS). Sleep Med 2020;76:89–97.
9. Buysse DJ. Sleep Health: can we define it? Does it matter? Sleep 2014;37(1):9–17.
10. Matricciani L, Paquet C, Fraysse F, et al. Sleep and cardiometabolic risk: a cluster analysis of actigraphy-derived sleep profiles in adults and children. Sleep 2021. https://doi.org/10.1093/sleep/zsab014.
11. Knutson KL, Phelan J, Paskow MJ, et al. The national sleep foundation's sleep health index. Sleep Health 2017;3(4):234–40.
12. Montag SE, Knutson KL, Zee PC, et al. Association of sleep characteristics with cardiovascular and metabolic risk factors in a population sample: the Chicago area sleep study. Sleep Health 2017; 3(2):107–12.
13. Asarnow LD, Mcglinchey E, Harvey AG. Evidence for a possible link between bedtime and change in body mass index. Sleep 2015;38(10):1523–7.
14. Olds TS, Maher CA, Matricciani L. Sleep duration or Bedtime ? Exploring the relationship between sleep habits and weight status and activity patterns. Sleep 2011;34(10):1299–307.

15. Knutson KL, Wu D, Patel SR, et al. Association between sleep timing , obesity , diabetes : the hispanic community health study/study of latinos (HCHS/SOL) cohort study. Sleep 2017;40(4):zsx014.

16. Baron KG, Reid KJ, Kim T, et al. Circadian timing and alignment in healthy adults: associations with BMI, body fat, caloric intake and physical activity. Int J Obes 2017;41(2):203–9.

17. Fritz J, Phillips AJK, Hunt LC, et al. Original article cross-sectional and prospective associations between sleep regularity and metabolic health in the hispanic community Health study/study of latinos. Sleep J 2020;44(4):zsaa218.

18. Milner CE, Cote KA. Benefits of napping in healthy adults: impact of nap length, time of day, age, and experience with napping. J Sleep Res 2009;18(2):272–81.

19. Cheungpasitporn W, Thongprayoon C, Srivali N, et al. The effects of napping on the risk of hypertension: a systematic review and meta-analysis. J Evid Based Med 2016;9(4):205–12.

20. Guo VY, Cao B, Wong CKH, et al. The association between daytime napping and risk of diabetes: a systematic review and meta-analysis of observational studies. Sleep Med 2017;37:105–12.

21. Zhong G, Wang Y, Tao TH, et al. Daytime napping and mortality from all causes, cardiovascular disease, and cancer: a meta-analysis of prospective cohort studies. Sleep Med 2015;16(7):811–9.

22. Pan Z, Huang M, Huang J, et al. Association of napping and all-cause mortality and incident cardiovascular diseases : a dose e response meta analysis of cohort studies. Sleep Med 2020;74:165–72.

23. Song C, Zhang R, Liao J, et al. Sleep quality and risk of coronary heart disease - a prospective cohort study from the English longitudinal study of ageing. Aging 2020;12(24):25005–19.

24. Kaneko H, Itoh H, Kiriyama H, et al. Restfulness from sleep and subsequent cardiovascular disease in the general population. Sci Rep 2020;10(1):19674.

25. Cortelli P, Lombardi C, Montagna P, et al. Baroreflex modulation during sleep and in obstructive sleep apnea syndrome. Auton Neurosci Basic Clin 2012;169(1):7–11.

26. Legramante JM, Marciani MG, Placidi F, et al. Sleep-related changes in baroreflex sensitivity and cardiovascular autonomic modulation. J Hypertens 2003;21(8):1555–61.

27. Herscovici S, Peer A, Papyan S, et al. Detecting REM sleep from the finger: an automatic REM sleep algorithm based on peripheral arterial tone (PAT) and actigraphy. Physiol Meas 2007;28(2):129–40.

28. Ren R, Covassin N, Zhang Y, et al. Interaction between slow wave sleep and obstructive sleep apnea in prevalent hypertension. Hypertension 2020;75:516–23.

29. Madsen P, Schmidt J, Wildschiødtz G, et al. Cerebral O2 metabolism and cerebral blood flow in humans during deep and rapid-eye-movement sleep. J Appl Physiol (1985) 1991;70(6):2597–601.

30. Hanak V, Somers VK. Cardiovascular and cerebrovascular physiology in sleep. In: Montagna P, Chokroverty S, editors. Handbook of clinical neurology. Elsevier; 2011. p. 315–25.

31. Braun A, Balkin T, Wesenten N, et al. Regional cerebral blood flow throughout the sleep-wake cycle. An H2(15)O PET study. Brain 1997;120(Pt. 7):1173–97.

32. Loos N, Grant DA, Wild J, et al. Sympathetic nervous control of the cerebral circulation in sleep. J Sleep Res 2005;14:275–83.

33. Bangash MF, Xie A, Skatrud JB, et al. Cerebrovascular response to arousal from NREM and REM sleep. Sleep 2008;31(3):321–7.

34. Kotajima F, Meadows GE, Morrell MJ, et al. Cerebral blood flow changes associated with fluctuations in alpha and theta rhythm during sleep onset in humans. J Physiol 2005;568(1):305–13.

35. Schmidt MH. The energy allocation function of sleep: a unifying theory of sleep, torpor, and continuous wakefulness. Neurosci Biobehavioral Rev 2014;47:122–53.

36. Borbély AA, Daan S, Wirz-Justice A, et al. The two-process model of sleep regulation: a reappraisal. J Sleep Res 2016;25(2):131–43.

37. Burgess HJ, Trinder J, Kim Y. Cardiac autonomic nervous system activity during presleep wakefulness and Stage 2 NREM sleep. J Sleep Res 1999;8(2):113–22.

38. Burgess HJ, Trinder J, Kim Y. Cardiac parasympathetic nervous system activity does not increase in anticipation of sleep. J Sleep Res 1996;5(2):83–9.

39. Somers V, Dyken M, Mark A, et al. Sympathetic-nerve activity during sleep in normal subjects. N Engl J Med 1993;328(5):303–7.

40. Bonnet MH, Arand DL. Heart rate variability: sleep stage, time of night, and arousal influences. Electroencephalogr Clin Neurophysiol 1997;102(5):390–6.

41. Silvani A. Physiological sleep-dependent changes in arterial blood pressure: central autonomic commands and baroreflex control. Clin Exp Pharmacol Physiol 2008;35(9):987–94.

42. Baharav A, Kotagal S, Gibbons V, et al. Fluctuations in autonomic nervous activity during sleep displayed by power spectrum analysis of heart rate variability. Neurology 1995;45(6):1183–7.

43. Murali N, Svatikova A, Somers V. Cardiovascular physiology and sleep. Front Biosci 2003;(27):636–52.

44. Guilleminault C, Pool P, Motta J, et al. Sinus arrest during REM sleep in young adults. N Engl J Med 1984;311:1006–10.

45. Dickerson LW, Huang AH, Thurnher MM, et al. Relationship between coronary hemodynamic

changes and the phasic events of rapid eye movement sleep. Sleep 1993;16(6):550–7.

46. Tobaldini E, Proserpio P, Sambusida K, et al. Preserved cardiac autonomic dynamics during sleep in subjects with spinal cord injuries. Sleep Med 2015;16(6):779–84.

47. Tobaldini E, Nobili L, Strada S, et al. Heart rate variability in normal and pathological sleep. Front Physiol 2013;4:294.

48. Baccelli G, Albertini R, Mancia G, et al. Central and reflex regulation of sympathetic vasoconstrictor activity to limb muscles during desynchronized sleep in the cat. Circ Res 1974; 35(4):625–35.

49. Mckinley MJ, Yao ST, Uschakov A, et al. The median preoptic nucleus: front and centre for the regulation of body fluid, sodium, temperature, sleep and cardiovascular homeostasis. Acta Physiol 2015;214(1):8–32.

50. Silvani A, Dampney RAL. Central control of cardiovascular function during sleep. Am J Physiol Heart Circ Physiol 2013;305(12):H1683–92.

51. Kondo H, Ozone M, Ohki N, et al. Association between heart rate variability, blood pressure and autonomic activity in cyclic alternating pattern during sleep. Sleep 2014;37(1):187–94.

52. Sforza E, Chapotot F, Lavoie S, et al. Heart rate activation during spontaneous arousals from sleep: effect of sleep deprivation. Clin Neurophysiol 2004; 115(11):2442–51.

53. Silvani A, Calandra-buonaura G, Dampney RAL, et al. Brain – heart interactions. Philos Trans A Math Phys Eng Sci 2016;374(2067):20150181.

54. Kuwaki T, Li A, Nattie E. State-dependent central chemoreception: a role of orexin. Respir Physiol Neurobiol 2010;173(3):223–9.

55. Van Cauter E, Polonsky KS, Scheen AJ. Roles of circadian rhythmicity and sleep in human glucose regulation. Endocr Rev 1997;18(5):716–38.

56. Saltiel AR, Kahn CR. Insulin signalling and the regulation of glucose and lipid metabolism. Nature 2001;414(6865):799–806.

57. Roh E, Kim MS. Brain regulation of energy metabolism. Endocrinol Metab 2016;31(4):519–24.

58. Saper CB, Cano G, Scammell TE. Homeostatic, circadian, and emotional regulation of sleep. J Comp Neurol 2005;493(1):92–8.

59. Messina G, Valenzano A, Moscatelli F, et al. Role of autonomic nervous system and orexinergic system on adipose tissue. Front Physiol 2017;8:137.

60. Favero G, Franceschetti L, Buffoli B, et al. Melatonin: protection against age-related cardiac pathology. Ageing Res Rev 2017;35:336–49.

61. Klimentova J, Cebova M, Barta A, et al. Effect of melatonin on blood pressure and nitric Oxide generation in rats with metabolic syndrome. Physiol Res 2016;65:373–80.

62. Peter JG, Fietze I. Physiology of the cardiovascular, endocrine and renal systems during sleep. Sleep Apnea 2006;35:29–36.

63. Buijs FN, Cazarez F, Basualdo MC, et al. The suprachiasmatic nucleus is part of a neural feedback circuit adapting blood pressure response. Neuroscience 2014;266:197–207.

64. Richards J, Diaz AN, Gumz ML. Clock genes in hypertension: novel insights from rodent models. Blood Press Monit 2014;19(5):249–54.

65. Dashti HS, Aslibekyan S, Scheer FA, et al. Clock genes explain a large proportion of phenotypic variance in systolic blood pressure and this control is not modified by environmental temperature. Am J Hypertens 2016;29(1):132–40.

66. Rüger M, Scheer F. Effects of circadian disruption on cardiometabolic system. Rev Endocr Metab Disord 2009;10(4):245–60.

67. Turek FW, Joshu C, Kohsaka A, et al. Obesity and metabolic syndrome in circadian clock mutant mice. Obesity 2005;308:1043–5.

68. Ivy JR, Oosthuyzen W, Peltz TS, et al. Glucocorticoids induce nondipping blood pressure by activating the thiazide-sensitive cotransporter. Hypertension 2016; 67(5):1029–37.

69. Ichikawa K. Changes in blood pressure and sleep duration in patients with blue light-blocking/yellow-tinted intraocular lens (CHUKYO study). Hypertens Res 2014;37(7):659–64.

70. Obayashi K, Saeki K, Iwamoto J, et al. Association between light exposure at night and nighttime blood pressure in the elderly independent of nocturnal urinary melatonin excretion. Chronobiol Int 2014;31(6):779–86.

71. Iwayama K, Kawabuchi R, Nabekura Y, et al. Exercise before breakfast increases 24-h fat oxidation in female subjects. PLoS One 2017;12(7): e0180472.

72. Van de Borne P, Nguyen H, Biston P, et al. Effects of wake and sleep stages on the 24-h autonomic control of blood pressure and heart rate in recumbent men. Am J Physiol 1994;266(2 Pt 2):H548–54.

73. Eguchi K, Kario K, Shimada K, et al. Circadian variation of blood pressure and neurohumoral factors during the acute phase of stroke. Clin Exp Hypertens 2002;24(1–2):109–14.

74. Brignole M, Auricchio A, Baron-Esquivias G, et al. 2013 ESC Guidelines on cardiac pacing and cardiac resynchronization therapy : addenda the Task Force on cardiac pacing and resynchronization therapy of the European Heart Rhythm Association(EHRA). Eur Heart J 2013;15(8):1070–118.

75. Gula LJ, Krahn AD, Skanes AC, et al. Clinical relevance of arrhythmias during sleep: guidance for clinicians. Heart 2004;90:347–52.

76. 2020 ESC Guidelines on sports cardiology and exercise in patients with cardiovascular disease the

Task Force on sports cardiology and exercise in patients with. Eur Heart J 2020;1–80.

77. Schwartz P, Crotti L, Insolia R. Long QT syndrome: from genetics to management. Circ Arrhythm Electrophysiol 2012;5(4):868–77.

78. Management of asymptomatic arrhythmias : a European heart rhythm association (EHRA) consensus document , endorsed by the heart failure association (HFA), heart rhythm society (HRS), asia pacific heart rhythm society (APHRS), Card Arrhythmia Society. Europace 2019;1–32.

79. Koehler U, Fus E, Grimm W, et al. Heart block in patients with obstructive sleep apnoea: pathogenetic factors and effects of treatment. Eur Resp J 1998;11(2):434–9.

80. Becker HF, Koehler U, Stammnitz A, et al. Heart block in patients with sleep apnoea. Thorax 1998; 53(Suppl 3):29–32.

81. Filchenko I, Bochkarev M, Kandinsky A. Continuous positive airway pressure therapy restores bradyarrhythmia with 10-second asystole in hypertensive obese patient with obstructive sleep apnea. Heart Rhythm Case Rep 2020;6(6):300–3.

82. Ludmer P, Selwyn A, Shook T, et al. Paradoxical vasoconstriction induced by acetylcholine in atherosclerotic coronary arteries. N Engl J Med 1986;315(17):1046–51.

83. Mancia G, Fagard R, Narkiewicz K, et al. 2013 ESH/ESC guidelines for the management of arterial hypertension: the Task Force for the management of arterial hypertension of the European Society of Hypertension (ESH) and of the European Society of Cardiology (ESC). Eur Heart J 2013;34(28): 2159–219.

84. Ben-Dov IZ, Kark JD, Ben-Ishay D, et al. Predictors of all-cause mortality in clinical ambulatory monitoring: unique aspects of blood pressure during sleep. Hypertension 2007;49(6):1235–41.

85. Marrocco-trischitta MM, Cremona G. Peripheral baroreflex and chemoreflex function after eversion carotid endarterectomy. J Vasc Surg 2013;58:136–45.

86. Rupprecht S, Finn S, Ehrhardt J, et al. Autonomic outcome is better after endarterectomy than after stenting in patients with asymptomatic carotid stenosis. J Vasc Surg 2021;64(4):975–84.

87. Nattie E, Li A. Central chemoreception in wakefulness and sleep: evidence for a distributed network and a role for orexin. J Appl Physiol (1985) 2010; 108(5):1417–24.

88. Mansukhani M, Wang S, Somers V. Chemoreflex physiology and implications for sleep apnea – insights from studies in humans. Exp Physiol 2015; 100(2):130–5.

89. Narkiewicz K, van de Borne PJH, Pesek Ca, et al. Selective potentiation of peripheral chemorelfex sensitivity in obstructive sleep apnea. Circulation 1999;99:1183–9.

90. Eugenín J, Larraín C, Zapata P. Plasticity of cardiovascular chemoreflexes after prolonged unilateral carotid body denervation: implications for its therapeutic use. Am J Physiol Heart Circ Physiol 2020; 318(5):H1325–36.

91. Dahan A, Nieuwenhuijs D, Teppema L. Plasticity of central Chemoreceptors : effect of bilateral carotid body resection on central CO 2 sensitivity. PLoS Med 2007;4(7):e239.

92. Manfredini R, Gallerani M, Boari B, et al. Morning preference in onset of symptomatic third-degree atrioventricular heart block. Chronobiol Int 2002; 19(4):785–91.

93. Guilleminault C, Connolly SJ, Winkle RA. Cardiac arrhythmia and conduction disturbances during sleep in 400 patients with sleep apnea syndrome. Am J Cardiol 1983;52(5):490–4.

94. Manfredini R, Gallerani M, Portaluppi F, et al. Relationships of the circadian rhythms of thrombotic, ischemic, hemorrhagic, and arrhythmic events to blood pressure rhythms. Ann N Y Acad Sci 1996; 783:141–58.

95. Manfredini R, Boari B, Smolensky M, et al. Circadian variation in stroke onset: identical temporal pattern in ischemic and hemorrhagic events. Chronobiol Int 2005;22(3):417–53.

96. Manfredini R, Gallerani M, Portaluppi F, et al. Chronobiological aspects of pulmonary thromboembolism. Int J Cardiol 1995;52(1):31–7.

97. Mehta R, Manfredini R, Hassan F, et al. Chronobiological patterns of acute aortic dissection. Circulation 2002;106(9):1110–5.

98. Smolensky M, Portaluppi F, Manfredini R, et al. Diurnal and twenty-four hour patterning of human diseases: cardiac, vascular, and respiratory diseases, conditions, and syndromes. Sleep Med Rev 2015;21:3–11.

99. Manfredini R, Portaluppi F, Boari B, et al. Circadian variation in onset of acute cardiogenic pulmonary edema is independent of patients' features and underlying pathophysiological causes. Chronobiol Int 2000;17(5):705–15.

100. Jones D, Bellomo R, Bates S, et al. Patient monitoring and the timing of cardiac arrests and medical emergency team calls in a teaching hospital. Intensive Care Med 2006;32(9): 1352–6.

101. Ramireddy A, Chugh H, Reinier K, et al. Sudden cardiac death during nighttime hours Archana. Heart Rhythm 2020. https://doi.org/10.1016/j.hrthm.2020.12.035.

102. Manfredini R, Gallerani M, Portaluppi F, et al. Circadian variation in the occurrence of paroxysmal supraventricular tachycardia in clinically healthy subjects. Chronobiol Int 1995;12(1):55–61.

103. Gami A, Olson E, Shen W, et al. Obstructive sleep apnea and the risk of sudden cardiac death: a

longitudinal study of 10,701 adults. J Am Collegue Cardiol 2013;62:610–6.

104. Gami AS, Howard DE, Olson EJ, et al. Day-night pattern of sudden death in obstructive sleep apnea. N Engl J Med 2005. https://doi.org/10.1056/NEJMoa041832.

105. Zucconi M, Ferri R. Assessment of sleep disorders and diagnostic procedures. Classification of sleep disorders. In: Sleep medicine textbook. European Sleep Research Society; 2014. p. 95–109.

106. Verdecchia P, Angeli F, Mazzotta G, et al. Ambulatory blood pressure monitoring day-night dip and early-morning surge in blood pressure prognostic implications. Hypertension 2012;60(1):34–43.

107. Kario K, Pickering T, Umeda Y, et al. Morning surge in blood pressure as a predictor of silent and clinical cerebrovascular disease in elderly hypertensives A prospective study. Circulation 2003;107:1401–6.

108. Palatini P, Reboldi G, Beilin LJ, et al. Predictive value of night-time heart rate for cardiovascular events in hypertension. the ABP-international study. Int J Cardiol 2013;168(2):1490–5.

109. Gupta A, Shukla G, Afsar M, et al. Prevention of new vascular events in patients with obstructive sleep apnea and stroke, using CPAP: a randomized controlled trial. Sleep Med 2015;16:S26.

110. Scheer F, Shea S. Human circadian system causes a morning peak in prothrombotic plasminogen activator inhibitor-1 (PAI-1) independent of the sleep/wake cycle. Blood 2014;123(4):590–3.

111. Pinotti M, Bertolucci C, Portaluppi F, et al. Daily and circadian rhythms of tissue factor Pathway inhibitor and factor VII activity. Arterioscler Thromb Vasc Biol 2005;25:646–9.

112. Tosur Z, Green D, De Chavez P, et al. The association between sleep characteristics and prothrombotic markers in a population based sample: Chicago area sleep study. Sleep Med 2014;15(8):973–8.

113. Grimaldi D, Carter JR, Cauter EV, et al. Adverse impact of sleep restriction and circadian misalignment on autonomic function in healthy young adults. Hypertension 2016;68(1):243–50.

114. Grimaldi D, Reid K, Papalambros N, et al. Autonomic dysregulation and sleep homeostasis in insomnia. Sleep 2020. https://doi.org/10.1093/sleep/zsaa274.

115. Li X, Sotres-Alvarez D, Gallo L, et al. Associations of sleep disordered breathing and insomnia with incident hypertension and diabetes: the hispanic community health study/study of latinos. Am J Respir Crit Care Med 2020. https://doi.org/10.1164/rccm.201912-2330OC.

116. Cholley-Roulleau M, Chenini S, Béziat S, et al. Restless legs syndrome and cardiovascular diseases: a case-control study. PLoS One 2017;12(4):e0176552.

117. Dean DA, Wang R, Jacobs DR, et al. A systematic assessment of the association of polysomnographic indices with blood pressure: the multiethnic study of atherosclerosis (MESA). Sleep 2015;38(4):587–96.

118. Cebrián S, Gimeno O, Orozco D, et al. Hypoglycaemia and somnambulism: a case report. Diabetes Metab 2012;38(6):574–5.

119. Ma C, Pavlova M, Liu Y, et al. Probable REM sleep behavior disorder and risk of stroke: a prospective study. Neurology 2017;88(19):1849–55.

120. Nordstrand S, Juvodden H, Viste R, et al. Obesity and other medical comorbidities among NT1 patients after the Norwegian H1N1 influenza epidemic and vaccination campaign. Sleep 2020;43(5):zsz277.

121. Barateau L, Chenini S, Evangelista E, et al. Clinical autonomic dysfunction in narcolepsy type 1. Sleep 2019;42(12):zsz187.

122. He Q, Sun H, Wu X, et al. Sleep duration and risk of stroke: a dose–response meta-analysis of prospective cohort studies. Sleep Med 2017;32:66–74.

123. Morris CJ, Purvis TE, Hu K, et al. Circadian misalignment increases cardiovascular disease risk factors in humans. Proc Natl Acad Sci U S A 2016;113(10):E1402–11.

124. Scheer FA, Hilton MF, Mantzoros CS, et al. Adverse metabolic and cardiovascular consequences of circadian misalignment. Proc Natl Acad Sci U S A 2009;106(11):4453–8.

125. McHill AW, Wright KP. Role of sleep and circadian disruption on energy expenditure and in metabolic predisposition to human obesity and metabolic disease. Obes Rev 2017;18:15–24.

126. During EH, Kawai M. The functions of sleep and the effects of sleep deprivation. Elsevier Inc; 2017.

127. Pigarev I. The visceral theory of sleep. Zh Vyssh Nerv Deiat Im I P Pavlova 2013;63(1):86–104.

128. Mensen A, Zhang Z, Qi M, et al. The occurrence of individual slow waves in sleep is predicted by heart rate. Sci Rep 2016;6:6–13.

129. Lavrova V, Busygina I, Pigarev I. The refection of cardiac activity on the electroencephalogram of cats in slow-wave sleep. Sensory Syst 2019;33(1):70–6.

130. Pigarev I, Pigareva M. Sleep and control of visceral functions. Russ J Physiol 2011;97(4):374–87.

131. Pigarev IN, Pigareva ML. Therapeutic effects of electrical Stimulation : interpretations and predictions based on the visceral theory of sleep. Front Neurosci 2018;12:10–2.

132. Iliff JJ, Wang M, Zeppenfeld DM, et al. Cerebral arterial pulsation drives paravascular CSF – interstitial fluid exchange in the murine brain. J Neurosci 2013;33(46):18190–9.

133. Lechinger J, Heib D, Gruber W, et al. Heartbeat-related EEG amplitude and phase modulations

from wakefulness to deep sleep: interactions with sleep spindles and slow oscillations. Psychophysiology 2015;52(11):1441–50.

134. Forouzanfar M, Baker FC, Colrain I, et al. Electroencephalographic slow-wave activity during sleep in different phases of blood pressure and respiration oscillations. Conf Proc IEEE Eng Med Biol Soc 2019;2019:2564–7.

135. Brindle RC, Duggan KA, Cribbet MR, et al. Cardiovascular stress reactivity and carotid intima-media thickness: the buffering role of slow-wave sleep. Psychosom Med 2018;80(3):301–6.

136. Kwon Y, Gadi SR, Shah NR, et al. Atrial fibrillation and objective sleep quality by slow wave sleep. J Atrial Fibrillation 2018;11(2):2031.

137. Xie L, Kang H, Xu Q, et al. Sleep drives metabolite clearance from the adult brain lulu. Science 2014; 342(6156):373–7.

138. Kim Y-K, Nam K II, Song J. The glymphatic system in diabetes-induced dementia. Front Neurol 2018; 9:867.

139. Hablitz LM, Vinitsky HS, Sun Q, et al. Increased glymphatic influx is correlated with high EEG delta power and low heart rate in mice under anesthesia. Sci Adv 2019;5:eaav5447.

140. Fallaize R, Carvalho-Wells AL, Tierney AC, et al. APOE genotype influences insulin resistance, apolipoprotein CII and CIII according to plasma fatty acid profile in the Metabolic Syndrome. Sci Rep 2017;7(1):6274.

141. Martínez-Martínez AB, Torres-Perez E, Devanney N, et al. Beyond the CNS: the many peripheral roles of APOE. Neurobiol Dis 2020;138: 104809.

142. Yesavage JA, Friedman L, Kraemer H, et al. Sleep/wake disruption in alzheimer's disease: APOE status and longitudinal course. J Geriatr Psychiatry Neurol 2004;17(1):20–4.

143. Badaut J, Copin J, Fukuda AM, et al. Increase of arginase activity in old apolipoprotein-E deficient mice under Western diet associated with changes in neurovascular unit. J Neuroinflammation 2012; 9(1):132–43.

144. Hirshkowitz M, Whiton K, Albert SM, et al. National sleep foundation's sleep time duration recommendations: methodology and results summary. Sleep Health 2015;1(1):40–3.

145. Ohayon M, Wickwire EM, Hirshkowitz M, et al. National Sleep Foundation's sleep quality recommendations: first report. Sleep Health 2017;3(1):6–19.

146. Hermida R, Ayala D, Mojón A, et al. Bedtime dosing of antihypertensive medications reduces cardiovascular risk in CKD. J Am Soc Nephrol 2011;22(12):2313–21.

147. Hermida R, Ayala D, Fernández J, et al. Administration-time differences in effects of hypertension medications on ambulatory blood pressure regulation. Chronobiol Int 2013;30(1–2):280–314.

148. Smolensky M, Hermida R, Geng Y-J. Chronotherapy of cardiac and vascular disease: timing medications to circadian rhythms to optimize treatment effects and outcomes. Curr Opin Pharmacol 2020;57:41–8.

149. Loloei S, Sepidarkish M, Heydarian A, et al. The effect of melatonin supplementation on lipid profile and anthropometric indices: a systematic review and meta-analysis of clinical trials. Diabetes Metab Syndr 2019;13(3):1901–10.

150. Baydas G, Yilmaz O, Celik S, et al. Effects of certain micronutrients and melatonin on plasma lipid, lipid peroxidation, and homocysteine levels in rats. Arch Med Res 2002;33(6):515–9.

151. Rahman M, Kwon H-S, Kim M-J, et al. Melatonin supplementation plus exercise behavior ameliorate insulin resistance, hypertension and fatigue in a rat model of type 2 diabetes mellitus. Biomed Pharmacother 2017;92:606–14.

152. Xu F, Xiao JZ, Shan LS, et al. Melatonin alleviates vascular calcification and ageing through exosomal miR-204/miR-211 cluster in a paracrine manner. J Pineal Res 2020;68:e12631.

153. Lu L, Ma J, Sun M, et al. Melatonin ameliorates MI-induced cardiac remodeling and apoptosis through a JNK/p53-dependent mechanism in diabetes mellitus. Oxid Med Cell Lobgev 2020;2020: 1535201.

154. Rosing BDR, Brakman P, et al. Blood fibrinolytic activity in man. Circulat Res 1970;27(1):171–84.

155. Reid KJ, Santostasi G, Baron KG, et al. Timing and intensity of light correlate with body weight in adults. PLoS One 2014;9(4):e92251.

156. Cheung IN, Zee PC, Shalman D, et al. Morning and evening blue-enriched light exposure alters metabolic function in normal weight adults. PLoS One 2016;11(5):e0155601.

157. Cordi MJ, Ackermann S, Rasch B. Effects of relaxing music on healthy sleep. Sci Data 2019;9:9079.

158. Grimaldi D, Papalambros NA, Zee PC, et al. Neurobiology of Disease Neurostimulation techniques to enhance sleep and improve cognition in aging. Neurobiol Dis 2020;141:104865.

159. Grimaldi D, Papalambros NA, Reid KJ, et al. Original article Strengthening sleep – autonomic interaction via acoustic enhancement of slow oscillations. Sleep J 2019;42(5):1–11.

160. Korkutata M, Saitoh T, Cherasse Y, et al. Neuropharmacology Enhancing endogenous adenosine A 2A receptor signaling induces slow-wave sleep without affecting body temperature and cardiovascular function. Neuropharmacology 2019;144: 122–32.

Sleep in Neurologic Disorders

Carlotta Mutti, MD, Francesco Rausa, MD, Liborio Parrino, MD, PhD*

KEYWORDS

• Neurological disorders • Epilepsy • Stroke • ALS • Sleep • Encephalitis • Neurodegeneration

KEY POINTS

- New-onset sleep disorders may herald subtle neurologic disorders such as autoimmune encephalitis and neurodegenerative disorders.
- Untreated sleep disorders frequently worsen the clinical outcome of patients with neurologic diseases and may interfere with the effectiveness of neurorehabilitative programs.
- Sleep evaluation should always be included in the workup of neurologic patients.

INTRODUCTION

Sleep is a complex brain state with fundamental relevance for cognitive functions, synaptic plasticity, brain resilience, and autonomic balance. Sleep pathologies may interfere with cerebral circuit organization, leading to negative consequences and favoring the development of neurologic disorders. Conversely, the latter can interfere with sleep functions. Accordingly, assessment of sleep quality is always recommended in the diagnosis of patients with neurologic disorders and during neurorehabilitation programs. This review investigates the complex interplay between sleep and brain pathologies, focusing on diseases in which the association with sleep disturbances is commonly overlooked and whereby major benefits may derive from their proper management.

SLEEP AND STROKE

Stroke is among the commonest cause of death worldwide; it can be strongly disabling in survivals and is associated with dramatic social and economic burden.[1] A relevant amount of sleep disorders, not limited to sleep-breathing disorders, may act as risk factors, and the relationship between stroke and sleep is multifaced. Untreated sleep disorders in patients with stroke may jeopardize learning mechanisms and impair the quality of neurorehabilitative processes.

The incidence of acute cerebrovascular infarction is modulated by well-known circadian rhythmicity, with approximately 25% of events occurring in the early morning hours.[2] Fibrinolytic capacity typically decreases in the morning, due to daily variation in plasminogen activator inhibitor-1 concentration and circadian changes in thrombosis mechanism.[3,4] Excessive amount/level of sleep fragmentation, as those affecting severe patients with obstructive sleep apnea (OSA), may lead to severe autonomic impact and higher risk for blood hypertension, overall promoting a higher risk for acute vascular events.[5] Moreover, sleep stages undergo multiple autonomic changes, moving from a parasympathetic predominance during nonrapid eye movement (NREM) sleep to a more irregular vegetative background during the last part of the night, when the prevailing REM sleep exerts relevant consequences on both blood pressure and heart rate.[6] Sleep-wake disorders due to circadian misalignment, such as shift work and circadian rhythm disorders, have also been associated with higher risk

Sleep Disorders Center, Department of Medicine and Surgery, Neurology Unit, University of Parma, Via Gramsci 14, Parma 43126, Italy
* Corresponding author.
E-mail address: liborio.parrino@unipr.it

Sleep Med Clin 16 (2021) 499–512
https://doi.org/10.1016/j.jsmc.2021.05.002
1556-407X/21/© 2021 Elsevier Inc. All rights reserved.

for hypertension and chronic inflammation,[7] 2 of the strongest risk factors for stroke, with the limitation in most of studies due to extreme variability with respect of dietary habits, lifestyle, or work stress.

Sleep quality and duration are essential to guarantee adequate metabolic balance and glucose tolerance,[8] and sleep fragmentation is a well-known risk factor for both diabetes, metabolic syndrome, and obesity. Sleep curtailment, independently from its cause, and specifically when slow wave sleep (SWS) duration is shortened, may lead to blood hypertension.[9] Sleep quality and depth in the first sleep cycles is also involved in modulating cortisol and norepinephrine fluctuations.[10]

Various manageable sleep disorders significantly increase the risk for stroke. In particular, OSA doubles the risk for acute stroke, increases the risk for stroke recurrence, and worsen neurologic outcome, whereas periodic leg movement disorder has been recently confirmed as independent risk factor for vascular events[11] and is associated with higher amount of white matter hyperintensities in neuroradiological investigations, a well-known radiological hallmark for small vessels diseases and incident stroke.[12] Complex mechanisms are involved in augmenting stroke risk among patients with OSA, including alterations of cerebrovascular reactivity, continuous stress due to intermittent hypoxia, thickening of carotid intima layer,[13] chronic low-grade inflammation, and augmented risk for paradoxic embolism in subjects presenting with patent foramen ovale.[14] A significant subgroup of patients with OSA, especially those suffering from marked obesity, may suffer from coexistent nocturnal hypoventilation syndrome (OHS), which is defined by a resting daytime arterial carbon dioxide tension (Pa_{CO_2}) of greater than or equal to 6 kPa, body mass index of greater than or equal to 30 kg/m², and the absence of an alternative cause of alveolar hypoventilation. Patients with OHS have higher mortality and morbidity compared with patients with OSA,[15] and the condition may promote progressive left atrial enlargement,[16] a relevant cardiogenic risk factor for stroke, and atrial fibrillation.[17,18]

Sleep macrostructure is variably compromised in poststroke patients, with changes ranging from decrease in SWS amount,[19] increased stage N1 of NREM sleep, and REM sleep curtailment.[20] Local slow wave activity dynamics in the periictal area had been interpreted as an electrophysiological measure for regional deafferentation,[21] frequently related to poorer functional outcome.

Poststroke Scenario

Sleep disorders may not only favor the first stroke occurrence but they may frequently complicate the poststroke scenario, with insomnia[22] and sleep-related breathing disorders[23] representing the most commonly described sequelae.

It is estimated that OSA affects around 70% of poststroke survivals.[24] Vulnerability to sleep stressors may help to predict the development of poststroke sleep disorders.[25] According to stroke severity and comorbidities different phenotypes for poststroke OSA have been proposed[26] and various quick-to-use prediction tolls had been developed to assess the risk for sleep apnea among patients with transient ischemic attacks or stroke, mostly derived by the validated STOP-BANG questionnaire (**Fig. 1**).[27,28]

Sleep apnea may be favored by the poststroke instability of neurologic and cardiorespiratory systems and, if untreated, may foster progression of chronic heart failure.[29] Patients already suffering from OSA may require periodic reassessment of their noninvasive ventilatory devices after an acute vascular episode, and central respiratory events may prevail over the obstructive ones due to changes in cardiovascular parameters and/or chemoreceptor sensitivity.[30] Finally psychotherapy-based approaches and acupuncture may help improve poststroke insomnia[31] with potential benefits on neurorehabilitation treatments.[32,33]

Summary

A comprehensive evaluation of the sleep profile should always be conducted both at first health screening level in high-risk cohorts and during the poststroke follow-up, to collect additional information, complementary to routine tests. Empowerment of sleep depth and continuity may have a supportive effect on the rehabilitative process.

SLEEP AND AMYOTROPHIC LATERAL SCLEROSIS

Amyotrophic lateral sclerosis (ALS) is a degenerative multisystemic neuromuscular disorder leading to progressive loss of voluntary movements control associated with variable neuropsychological and cognitive symptoms. The metabolic disruption of several proteins, including TDP-43 (TAR-DNA binding protein 43 kDa) and microtubule-associated tau protein, plays a pathogenetic role in the disease.[34,35] In recent years growing attention has been dedicated to the non-motor consequences of the pathology, beyond the classic

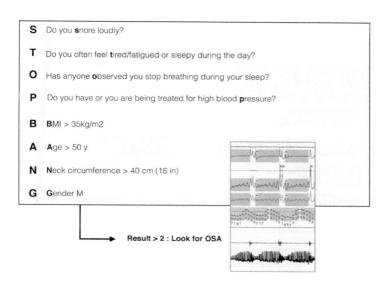

Fig. 1. STOP-BANG questionnaire: a screening test for OSA.

motor weakness[34] and including sleep disturbances.

Sleep disorders reported in patients with ALS include circadian rhythm disorders, sleep fragmentation, sleep-related movement disorders, and sleep breathing disorders.[36] ALS could lead to sleep disturbances including neuropsychological issues (anxiety, depression), cramps, muscle pain, restless leg syndrome (RLS), nocturnal hypoventilation, and sleep apneas.[37] Furthermore, direct damage of key regions of sleep regulation (suprachiasmatic nucleus, thalamus, prefrontal cortex) has been demonstrated.[38]

Around 60% of patients with ALS reported bad sleep quality and/or excessive daytime sleepiness, and poor sleepers suffer from more disabling daytime consequences including anxiety, depression, and cognitive impairment.[39] So far sleep disorders in patients with ALS have been explored using self-assessed questionnaires, whereas only few investigations provide objective data based on instrumental findings.[36] Compared with healthy controls, affected subjects presented reduced sleep efficiency and shortened total sleep time, frequent awakening, and more time spent in light NREM sleep stages.[40–42] Sleep instability, mirrored by CAP rate, is reduced and relevant decrease of CAP subtypes A1 is appreciable, hampering the build-up of SWS.[43] Depletion of physiologic graphoelements of NREM sleep and reduction and fragmentation of SWS had also been described in the most severe clinical phenotypes,[44,45] revealing the potential significance of abnormal sleep features as prognostic factors. Heart rate variability, a validated biomarker for dysautonomia, is altered throughout all sleep stages.[43] Genetic ALS phenotypes are at higher risk for the development of sleep-wake disturbances and daytime sleepiness compared with sporadic ones.[39]

The first phase of the disease, before respiratory function impairment, is usually characterized by sleep fragmentation, insomnia, fatigue, and daytime sleepiness. Motor disability favors the development of sleep-related motor disorders such as RLS or cramps.[46] Forced immobilization and sarcopenia may exacerbate both disturbances. As the neurodegenerative process evolves, major disabilities emerge due to nocturnal hypoventilation and other sleep-related breathing disorders may appear, strongly contributing to poor sleep and lower quality of life (Fig. 2). OSA is prevalent among patients with spinal ALS, whereas bulbar patients are more protected by the early development of tongue atrophy.[47] Nocturnal hypoventilation may develop in both patients with spinal as well as bulbar ALS, and scheduled investigations, including transcutaneous capnometry, are recommended for an early diagnose of nocturnal hypoventilation, as symptoms may be blurry and delayed.[48] Diaphragmatic weakness progressively leads to carbon monoxide accumulation, firstly limited to REM sleep stages (a sleep stage when diaphragm is the major determinant for ventilation), then progressively worsen and involve also NREM sleep stages. Numerous studies demonstrated that nocturnal noninvasive ventilation in patents with ALS improve survivals, quality of life, and sleep.[49]

Because of the progressive nature of the ALS, follow-up programs assessing optimal mask fitting, promoting adherence to treatment, and ensuring the synchrony between ventilator and

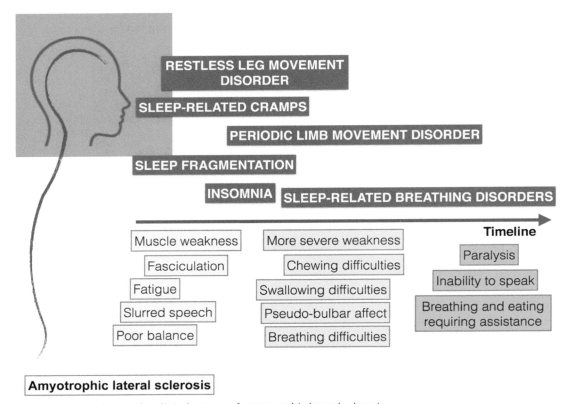

Fig. 2. Sleep disorders in the clinical course of amyotrophic lateral sclerosis.

patient's breathing dynamics are mandatory.[46] Several motor tests had been proposed as screening tolls to allow timely recognition of nocturnal hypoventilation: sniff nasal inspiratory pressure and base excess (with threshold around 2.3) seem robust predictors for "spinal patients," whereas lack of evidences of these or other tests in the "bulbar" phenotypes.[50]

Summary

The sleep clinician should always be included in the multidisciplinary evaluation of this severe neurodegenerative disorder. The clinical course of ALS may deal with different sleep disorders ranging from sleep fragmentation to sleep-related movement or breathing disorders. Scheduled evaluations by sleep experts are required to ensure prompt management of the ongoing ALS conditions.

SLEEP AND AUTOIMMUNE ENCEPHALITIS

Sleep disorders are common among patients with autoimmune encephalitis (AE) but their presence is frequently underestimated due to concomitant severe neurologic issues.[51] Numerous sleep

disorders may occur in patients with autoimmune encephalitis, including sleep fragmentation, hypersomnia, NREM parasomnia, sleep-breathing disorders, REM-behavior disorder (RBD), and others.[51]

AE diagnosis is mainly focused on clinical, radiological, and laboratory findings, with only minor attention dedicated to sleep features analysis, excluding antiimmunoglobulin-like cell adhesion molecule 5 (IgLON5) encephalitis. The latter is a rare AE associated with tau deposition in the brainstem and hypothalamus[52] and with distinctive clinical aspects characterized by excessive daytime sleepiness, sleep fragmentation, irregular jerks, periodic limb movements during sleep and drowsiness, dream enactment, sleep hallucinations, sleep breathing disorders (apneic episodes and stridor), enuresis, disorders of arousal, shouting and vocalization, and abnormal purposeful sleep behaviors (with eyes closed and closely resembling daytime activities) with no dream recall.[53] Coexistent neurologic manifestations include bulbar signs, gait imbalance, and cognitive decline, whereas fewer cases present with other signs such as movement disorders, Huntington-like symptoms, or fever.[54,55] Anatomic targets of the pathologic process in IgLON5 disease include brainstem, hypothalamus, ventral medulla, and nucleus ambiguous, all areas involved in breathing control, vocal cord motility, and NREM/REM sleep dynamics.[56] One of the distinctive features of the disease is the loss of the normal complexity of NREM sleep stages, and common rules to score can be impossible to apply. "Undifferentiated NREM sleep" and "poorly structured N2" had been proposed to allow video-polysomnographic scoring of anti-IgLON5 patients. Interestingly sleep abnormalities are most prominent in the first part of the night and gradually improve during the night, when a more recognizable and "conventional" (even if "delayed") stage N3 can be appreciated. Total sleep time is usually preserved, scant K-complexes and spindles are still recognizable during poorly structured N2, and circadian sleep-wake alternation is partially preserved.

Because of the absence of clear-cut inflammatory infiltrates, poor response to immunotherapy, and massive tau deposition, debate is still ongoing on the autoimmune or neurodegenerative nature of anti-IgLON.[57]

Other AE commonly associated with sleep disorders include anti-N-methyl-D-aspartate-receptor encephalitis (insomnia, confusional arousals), anti-AMPA (insomnia or hypersomnia), anti-LGI1 (insomnia, RBD), anti-CASPR2 (insomnia), anti-Ma2 (narcolepsy), and anti-Hu (nocturnal hypoventilation).[51]

The scenario is far from being comprehensive, hence in many cases sleep symptoms are overshadowed by concomitant neurologic or autonomic disorders. Investigation on new-onset sleep pathologies is rarely explored and video-polysomnographic recording is exceptionally accomplished. Even less is known regarding chronic consequences of AE on sleep, making it particularly difficult to estimate the reciprocal effect between AE and sleep.

Summary

AEs perturb sleep by means of numerous mechanisms involving direct pathologic damage by inflammatory cascades, drug side effects, predisposing comorbidities, genetic background, and deafferentation/disconnection syndromes. Longitudinal wide-sample studies, including instrumental investigations, are required to evaluate the impact of these disorders on sleep and wakefulness. Clinicians should always emphasize night symptoms and explore sleep recordings in patients with AE, as their recognition may shed light on the disease processing and dynamics even when conventional approaches may be uninformative.

SLEEP AND EPILEPSY

Epilepsy networks and sleep circuits are reciprocally embedded in multiple fashions. Continuous electroencephalogram (EEG) data provide some novel insights regarding the nonstochastic timing of seizure relapse, strongly driven by circadian rhythm.[58]

At night, the "sleep-promoting systems" gradually prevail on the "wake-promoting systems" leading to the construction of NREM sleep. The hippocampus fires with specific high-frequency strongly synchronized bursts ($\sim$80–120 Hz), named ripples, necessary for memory consolidation processes.[59]

Multisynaptic mechanisms promote the switch of the thalamocortical circuits from a tonic firing mode to an oscillatory "burst-firing" mode, which may appear at the surface-EEG as either spindles or delta, depending on the degree of membrane polarization/hyperpolarization.[60] NREM sleep is physiologically populated by infraslow oscillations, which are strongly synchronized with faster EEG activities.[61] In line with this framework NREM sleep texture includes periodic fluctuations, the cyclic alternating pattern (CAP), the electrophysiological hallmark of NREM sleep instability, and resilience.[62] Specifically, CAP subtype A1, composed of highly synchronizing patterns, enhances the thalamocortical oscillatory mode, building a permissive framework for highly synchronized activities to occur (eg, generalized epileptiform discharges).[63]

According to these aspects, sleep may promote epileptogenesis through multiple mechanisms, varying according to the epilepsy syndrome and including (1) the facilitatory effect of thalamocortical firing mode on the spreading of generalized spike and wave phenomena among idiopathic generalized epilepsies; (2) the remodulation of the hippocampal firing mode during NREM sleep, involved in the increased spike rate within the hippocampus and in the enlargement of the epileptiform field in mesial temporal lobe epilepsies (MTLE); and (3) the activation of "pathologic arousal reactions" in the sleep-related hypermotor epilepsy (SHE).[64,65] Pathologic fast ripples (200–600 Hz) have been proposed as electrical biomarkers for MTLE.[66] Overall EEG paroxysmal events take place mostly during transitional sleep states and periods of unstable sleep reflected by the higher global amount of EEG paroxysms during CAP compared with non-CAP sleep (**Fig. 3**).[67] Therefore, numerous NREM sleep mechanisms may promote the appearance and/or the spreading of paroxysmal activities. Both major episodes and minor events in SHE show a

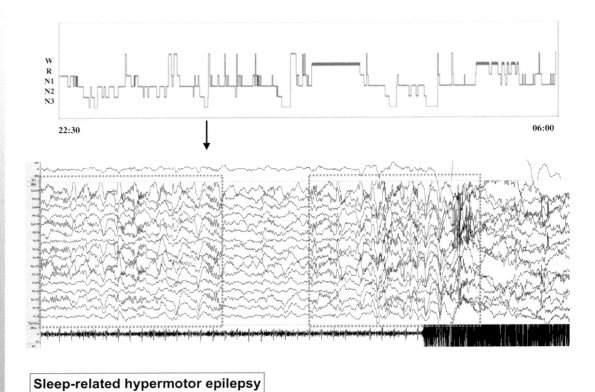

W
R
N1
N2
N3

22:30　　　　　　　　　　　　　　　　　　　　　　　　　　06:00

Sleep-related hypermotor epilepsy

Fig. 3. Paroxysmal arousal driven by NREM sleep instability during stage N3. Note slow wave sleep fragmentation.

dramatic association with the slow EEG components of phase A subtypes, K-complexes, and delta bursts,[68] known as "dysosmia" pattern.[69]

With respect to alertness and vigilance epileptic patients frequently complain of excessive daytime sleepiness and unrefreshing sleep,[70] related to a possible compensatory excessive amount of SWS, SWS fragmentation due to higher CAP fluctuations,[71] and increased duration of CAP sequences.[72]

Because sleep plays a role in consolidating memory and promoting plasticity, its fragmentation may compromise the efficacy of NREM-dependent cognitive mechanisms.[73] At the same time, in a vicious circle perspective, the empowerment of sleep instability, induced by the excess of epileptiform discharges, may booster seizure relapse. The most extreme scenario is the one where epileptiform discharges cover almost the entire brain rhythm during sleep, derailing it into the continuous slow-wave activity (SWA) during sleep or electrical status epilepticus in sleep.[74] The latter is a rare childhood-related disorder of either genetic or structural cause,[75] leading to cognitive regression and impressive NREM activation of epileptiform discharges during sleep.[76] The

nearly continuous ongoing epileptiform activity does not allow for memory consolidation process to occur, imposing severe cognitive disturbances.[77]

Epilepsy and Sleep Disorders

The relationship between sleep and epilepsy is frequently complicated due to potential coexistence of other (commonly overlooked) pathologies, including sleep breathing disorders, sleep-related movement disorders, insomnia, circadian rhythm disorders, and parasomnia.[78] In particular the relationship between SHE and NREM sleep parasomnias had been widely discussed. For sleep clinicians the differential diagnosis is highly challenging also because scalp EEG recording and brain MRI are frequently uninformative. So far, most studies seek for the distinctive features of the 2 conditions. However, the 2 entities show impressive similarities from a clinical, pathogenetic, and instrumental point of view, finding a common trail in the polysomnographic metrics.[71,73] The disorders may actually coexist in the same patient and family, probably sharing common genetic predisposition.[79] The hypothesized double-face nature of SHE and NREM parasomnia can extend the common therapeutic approaches. Carbamazepine at low dosage and single bedtime administration is still the first-line therapy for patients with SHE and possibly NREM parasomnia. Various antiepileptic drugs including lacosamide, oxcarbazepine, or topiramate may be used as either add-on or second-line monotherapy, and interesting alternatives include nicotine patch or fenofibrate, both influencing in distinct ways the activity of acetylcholine receptor.[80,81] All cases of drug-resistant nocturnal epilepsy should undergo complete presurgical evaluation and may reach adequate control of the disease with lesion (frequently focal cortical dysplasia) removal, especially when the lesion is located in the frontal lobe.[82] Accordingly coexistent sleep pathologies required adequate treatment when coexisting with epileptic syndromes or NREM parasomnias.[83,84]

Summary

Given the detrimental role of paroxysmal discharges on NREM sleep-related brain plasticity processes and, at the same time, the promoting role of sleep instability toward seizures generation and recurrence, it is surprising that sleep assessment is not part of the routinely diagnostic workup for epileptic patients. Coexistent sleep-related disorders may fuel aberrant circuits, triggering increasing intern levels of instability.[71] Poor sleep quality and daytime sleepiness are common in patients suffering from epilepsy, affecting seizure frequency and drug-resistance development.[70] Sleep and epilepsy are to consider as bad fellows, and the evaluation of their unlucky embedment is mandatory among patients suffering from epilepsy.

SLEEP AND NEURODEGENERATIVE DISORDERS

Subjects with neurodegenerative diseases show common features in the sleep texture: sleep fragmentation, loss of SWS and REM sleep, drop of sleep efficiency, increase of light sleep, and multiple nocturnal awakenings.[85] Given the early appearance of sleep disturbances in the clinical course of numerous neurodegenerative disorders, their recognition and treatment may favor a timely diagnosis and reduce the caregiver burden.[86] As a result of poor sleep, many patients develop excessive daytime sleepiness and rapid progression of cognitive impairment. Moreover, patients with neurodegenerative disorders suffering from untreated sleep disturbances are at higher risk for

falls, are affected by lower quality of life, and may be easily institutionalized.[87,88]

Sleep and Alzheimer Disease

The patients with Alzheimer disease frequently suffer from circadian misalignment, insomnia, fragmented, and superficial sleep. Moreover, the SWA decline within the prefrontal cortex induces malfunctioning of the hippocampal-cortical loop necessary for NREM-sleep–dependent memory consolidation.[89]

Recently, a close relationship between AD and OSA has been documented.[90] Both conditions share a progressive accumulation of β-amyloid in the brain within a framework of chronic low-grade inflammation and oxidative stress (**Fig. 4**). Apnea-related intermittent hypoxia fuels β-secretase activity, enhancing amyloid synthesis and accelerating AD pathology.[91,92] Hence, identification and treatment of overlooked sleep-breathing disorders in this cohort may slow the degeneration process.

Common sleep disorders may change their "aspect" in patients with AD. In particular, nighttime agitation or sundowning may become an unusual manifestation of an RLS.[93] This consideration warrants attention, as many drugs commonly used to treat nocturnal restlessness, such as antipsychotic medications, may worsen the clinical manifestations of RLS.

Management of sleep disturbances in patients with AD is challenging for sleep specialists, as benzodiazepines may enhance cognitive impairment,[94] whereas antidepressants may promote iatrogenic REM-behavior disorder.[95] Recommended approaches for sleep disturbances in patients with AD include cognitive behavioral therapy, light therapy, melatonin, and structured limb exercise. The use of the orexin receptor antagonist Suvorexant in patients with AD with insomnia has provided encouraging results.[96]

Sleep and Parkinson Disease

Sleep disorders are common prodromal manifestations in patients with Parkinson disease (PD) and include RBD, insomnia, RLS, OSA, circadian rhythm disorders, and excessive daytime sleepiness (EDS). These disturbances may sometimes coexist in the same patient.

RBD is characterized by repetitive episodes of dream enactment (sleep-related vocalization and/or complex motor behaviors) occurring during REM sleep.[97] Untreated RBD may lower quality of life and increase the risk for nocturnal injuries. Pathology of RBD is deeply embedded with alpha-synucleinopathy dynamics, and the condition is a

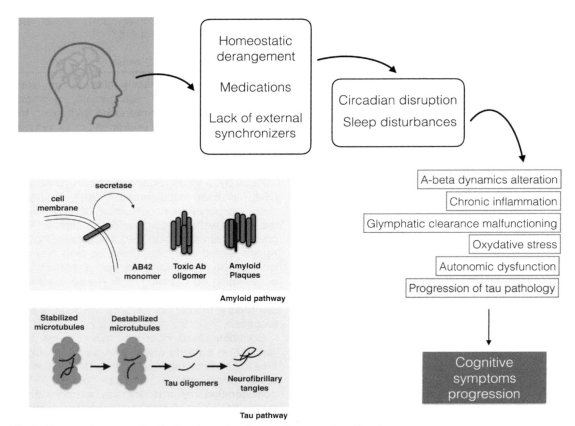

Fig. 4. Sleep-wake anomalies in the dynamic of neurodegenerative disorders.

risk factor for PD, multiple system atrophy (MSA), and dementia with Lewy body disease.[98] It is estimated that 25% to 58% of patients with PD and virtually all patients with MSA suffer from RBD.[99,100] Risk for conversion is higher among patients with RBD with microstructural non-REM sleep anomalies, such as a severe reduction of CAP fluctuations.[101] An interesting parallelism between the progressive drop of CAP rate, first involving subtypes A1, and the gradual neuropathological damage described in the Braak staging (from brainstem to rostral areas) had also been suggested.[101] Various medications including selective serotonin reuptake inhibitors, venlafaxine, tricyclic antidepressants, monoamine oxidase inhibitors, mirtazapine, and β-blockers may induce or worsen RBD.[102] RBD management is basically symptomatic and requires the avoidance of triggers, bedroom safety setting, and high dosage of melatonin (3–12 mg) and/or clonazepam (0.5–2 mg), the latter being associated with higher risk for cognitive impairment and OSA aggravation.[103]

Insomnia in patients with PD may be favored by coexistent motor (tremor, dystonia, restlessness) and nonmotor (mood disorders, nocturia) symptoms, often requiring tailored approaches.[104] Coexistent circadian misalignment may worsen the extent of sleep fragmentation, sometimes exacerbated by the usage of dopaminergic medications, which can reduce endogenous melatonin secretion.[105]

Untreated sleep disorders may increase the severity of cognitive and motor manifestation of PD.[106] Recent investigations highlighted the existence of unusual mechanisms sustaining the development of EDS in patients with PD, including the derailment of REM-on circuits, as demonstrated by the unexpected sleep-onset rapid eye movement period, the electrophysiological biomarkers of narcolepsy, at electrophysiological examination.[107]

Summary

Sleep is highly important in the context of neurodegeneration, and sleep disorders may worsen clinical impact in patients with neurodegenerative disorders.

SLEEP, HEADACHE, AND TRAUMATIC BRAIN INJURY: THE ROLE OF THE GLYMPHATIC SYSTEM

In 2012 Iliff and colleagues[108] discovered a dispose of waste mechanism in the central nervous system (CNS). This brain-wide fluid transport pathway was named "glymphatic" system, through which 40% to 80% of soluble proteins and metabolites are thought to be removed. The term "glymphatic" is derived from the functional similarities with the lymphatic system and by its dependence on glial water flux. This clearance system is a unique paravascular tunnel system necessary to shift soluble proteins and metabolites from the CNS, including neurotoxic compounds such as amyloid-β and tau.[109] The system works on dynamics of arterial pulsation and is supported by the astroglial water transport via the aquaporin-4 (AQP4) water channel.[110] Further roles of the glymphatic system include brain-wide distribution of important molecules such as glucose, amino acids, lipids, growth factors, and various neuromodulators.[109] The glymphatic system physiologically undergoes homeostatic regulation, increasing its activity up to 90% during sleep.[111] Sleep increases the volume of the brain extracellular space, which supports more rapid diffusion of metabolites and proteins between perivascular compartments. Therefore, sleep plays a supportive role on the CNS clearance through the glymphatic pathways.[109]

Growing evidences highlight the importance of the glymphatic system in manyfold neurologic disorders including AD, stroke, epilepsy, trauma brain injury (TBI), and headache.

Headache

It is estimated that around 48% to 74% of patients with migraine and 26% to 72% of patients with tension-type headaches recognize "lack of sleep" as a headache trigger.[112–114] Sleep deprivation and fragmentation can thus precipitate headache and foster its chronicization.[115] At the same time, patients affected by headache frequently complain of poor sleep quality, daytime sleepiness, and fatigue[116] and of various sleep disorders including insomnia, RLS, and NREM sleep parasomnias.[117] Sleep can interrupt a headache attack, and, vice-versa, intense cephalalgia can disturb sleep.[118] A recent study showed a relation between sleep disruption and lowered pain tolerance.[119] Serotonin (5-HT), a key molecule in sleep regulation, also influences human mood and central nociceptive pathways: reduced serotonin levels can foster pain but can also alter the sleep structure.[120] Certain types of headache are related to distinct sleep stages: cluster headaches and migraine are usually triggered by REM sleep, and hypnic headaches usually occur after 1 to 3 hours of sleep.[121] Moreover, there is evidence that arousal oscillations, expressed by CAP parameters, decrease in patients with migraine without aura.[122]

Migraine

Insomnia is the most common sleep disorder in patients with migraine, and the relationship seems bidirectional.[116] The increase in liquoral peptide concentration (glucagon-related peptide [GCRP], pituitary adenylate cyclase-activating peptide [PACAP]) is essential in the attack development, and newest therapies for migraine target on these pathways.[123] Cortical spreading depression (CSD) is the prototypical mechanism of migraine, characterized by a slowly spreading wave of neural activity alternating short excitatory periods to long-lasting inhibition.[124] In animal models CSD can reversibly hamper communication throughout the paravascular space, resulting in a transient glymphatic system impairment[125] and accumulation of GCRP and PACAP.[110] A single wave of CSD induces a 30-minute long complete closure of the paravascular space.[125] This blockage favors cortical hyperexcitability, increasing the risk for further migraine attacks or episodes of longer duration.[125–127]

Traumatic Brain Injury

Sleep-wake disturbances are frequent in patients with TBI.[128] Hypersomnolence appears frequently as the first posttraumatic sleep disturbance, and it is commonly followed by long-term chronic insomnia and sleep fragmentation.[129] The term "pleiosomnia" has been suggested to describe the need for additional sleep time (mean around 2 hours) in patients experiencing posttraumatic hypersomnia.[130] In the initial posttraumatic period, several polysomnographic indexes (spectral changes, SWS, coherence index) may be used to estimate trauma severity and prognosis.[131] A reduction in sleep efficiency, increased number of arousals, and sleep fragmentation are also evident in TBI.[132] The presence of untreated sleep disturbances may delay the recovery from trauma.[133] Different mechanisms are hypothesized to be at the basis of sleep disturbances after TBI: impaired production and secretion of melatonin, damage of the hypothalamic cells secreting orexin or of key areas involved in the sleep-wake regulatory process, and disruption of hormonal systems.[134] Finally, posttraumatic sleep disorders may exaggerate TBI consequences due to breakdown of the glymphatic system. TBI may lead to glymphatic pathways impairment indirectly, affecting sleep-wake cycle regularity or more directly, promoting a dislocation of AQP4, essential for paravascular drainage of toxic molecules. TBI is associated with tau deposition within the brain and increases the risk of an early development of dementia.[135–138] To what extent impairment of the glymphatic system and coexistent sleep disturbances are relevant for posttraumatic neurodegeneration remains an open question.

CLINICS CARE POINTS

- Sleep health mirrors brain health: do not forget to investigate sleep habits and quality during routine neurologic evaluation.
- Sleep is necessary for cognition and motor learning.
- Untreated sleep disorders should be handled, as they may affect the clinical outcome of neurologic patients.
- Sleep circuits are deeply entangled with epileptiform networks: sleep evaluation is strongly recommended for patients with epilepsy.
- Polysomnography could represent a noninvasive biomarker to detect prodromal neurodegeneration.

ACKNOWLEDGMENTS

None.

DISCLOSURE

The authors have nothing to disclose.

REFERENCES

1. Feigin VL, Forouzanfar MH, Krishnamurthi R, et al. Global and regional burden of stroke during 1990-2010: findings from the Global Burden of Disease Study 2010. Lancet 2014;383:245–54.

2. Fink JN, Kumar S, Horkan C, et al. The stroke patient who woke up: clinical and radiological features, including diffusion and perfusion MRI. Stroke 2002;33(4):988–93.

3. Scheer FAJL, Shea SA. Human circadian system causes a morning peak in prothrombotic plasminogen activator inhibitor-1 (PAI-1) independent of the sleep/wake cycle. Blood 2014;123(4):590–3.

4. Andreotti F, Kluft C. Circadian variation of fibrinolytic activity in blood. Chronobiol Int 1991;8:336–51.

5. Staats R, Barros I, Fernandes D, et al. The importance of sleep fragmentation on the hemodynamic dipping in obstructive sleep apnea patients. Front Physiol 2020;11:104.

6. Murali NS, Svatikova A, Somers VK. Cardiovascular physiology and sleep. Front Biosci 2003;8:s636–52.

7. Morris CJ, Purvis TE, Mistretta J, et al. Circadian misalignment increases C-reactive protein and blood pressure in chronic shift workers. J Biol Rhythms 2017;32(2):154–64.

8. Broussard JL, Ehrmann DA, Van Cauter E, et al. Impaired insulin signaling in human adipocytes after experimental sleep restriction: a randomized, crossover study. Ann Intern Med 2012;157(8):549–57.

9. Javaheri S, Zhao YY, Punjabi NM, et al. Slow-wave sleep is associated with incident hypertension: the sleep heart health study. Sleep 2018;41(1):zsx179.

10. Grimaldi D, Reid KJ, Papalambros NA, et al. Autonomic dysregulation and sleep homeostasis in insomnia. Sleep 2020;9:zsaa274.

11. Bassetti CLA, Randerath W, Vignatelli L, et al. EAN/ERS/ESO/ESRS statement on the impact of sleep disorders on risk and outcome of stroke. Eur Respir J 2020;55(4):1901104.

12. Boulos MI, Murray BJ, Muir RT, et al. Periodic limb movements and white matter hyperintensities in first-ever minor stroke or high-risk transient ischemic attack. Sleep 2017;40(3):zsw080.

13. López-Cano C, Rius F, Sánchez E, et al. The influence of sleep apnea syndrome and intermittent hypoxia in carotid adventitial vasa vasorum. PLoS One 2019;14(2):e0211742.

14. Arboix A. Cardiovascular risk factors for acute stroke: risk profiles in the different subtypes of ischemic stroke. World J Clin Cases 2015;3(5):418–29.

15. Castro-Anon O, de Llano LAP, Sanchez SDIF, et al. Obesity-hypoventilation syndrome: increased risk of death over sleep apnea syndrome. PLoS One 2015;10:e0117808.

16. Al-Khadra Y, Darmoch F, Alkhatib M, et al. Risk of left atrial enlargement in obese patients with obesity-induced hypoventilation syndrome vs obstructive sleep apnea. Ochsner J 2018;18(2):136–40.

17. Tokunaga K, Koga M, Yoshimura S, et al, for the SAMURAI Study Investigators. Left atrial size and ischemic events after ischemic stroke or transient ischemic attack in patients with nonvalvular atrial fibrillation. Cerebrovasc Dis 2020;49(6):619–24.

18. Trotti LM, Rye DB, De Staercke C, et al. Elevated C-reactive protein is associated with severe

periodic leg movements of sleep in patients with restless legs syndrome. Brain Behav Immun 2012;26(8):1239–43.

19. Terzoudi A, Vorvolakos T, Heliopoulos I, et al. Sleep architecture in stroke and relation to outcome. Eur Neurol 2009;61:16–22.

20. Duss SB, Seiler A, Schmidt MH, et al. The role of sleep in recovery following ischemic stroke: a review of human and animal data. Neurobiol Sleep Circadian Rhythms 2016;2:94–105.

21. Poryazova R, Huber R, Khatami R, et al. Topographic sleep EEG changes in the acute and chronic stage of hemispheric stroke. J Sleep Res 2015;24:54–65.

22. Baylan S, Griffiths S, Grant N, et al. Incidence and prevalence of post-stroke insomnia: a systematic review and meta-analysis. Sleep Med Rev 2020; 49:101222.

23. Brown DL, He K, Kim S, et al. Prediction of sleep-disordered breathing after stroke. Sleep Med 2020;75:1–6.

24. Johnson KG, Johnson DC. Frequency of sleep apnea in stroke and TIA patients: a meta- analysis. J Clin Sleep Med 2010;6:131–7.

25. Kalmbach DA, Anderson JR, Drake CL. The impact of stress on sleep: pathogenic sleep reactivity as a vulnerability to insomnia and circadian disorders. J Sleep Res 2018;27(6):e12710.

26. Schütz SG, Lisabeth LD, Shafie-Khorassani F, et al. Clinical phenotypes of obstructive sleep apnea after ischemic stroke: a cluster analysis. Sleep Med 2019;60:178–81.

27. Boulos MI, Colelli DR, Vaccarino SR, et al. Using a modified version of the "STOP-BANG" questionnaire and nocturnal oxygen desaturation to predict obstructive sleep apnea after stroke or TIA. Sleep Med 2019;56:177–83.

28. Katzan IL, Thompson NR, Uchino K, et al. A screening tool for obstructive sleep apnea in cerebrovascular patients. Sleep Med 2016;21:70–6.

29. Dharia SM, Brown LK. Epidemiology of sleep-disordered breathing and heart failure: what drives what. Curr Heart Fail Rep 2017;14(5):351–64.

30. De Paolis F, Colizzi E, Milioli G, et al. Acute shift of a case of moderate obstructive sleep apnea syndrome towards one of severe central sleep apnea syndrome after an ischemic stroke. Sleep Med 2012;13(6):763–6.

31. Lowe A, Bailey M, O'Shaughnessy T, et al. Treatment of sleep disturbance following stroke and traumatic brain injury: a systematic review of conservative interventions. Disabil Rehabil 2020;11: 1–13.

32. Fulk G, Duncan P, Klingman KJ. Sleep problems worsen health-related quality of life and participation during the first 12 months of stroke rehabilitation. Clin Rehabil 2020;34(11):1400–8.

33. Moon HI, Yoon SY, Jeong YJ, et al. Sleep disturbances negatively affect balance and gait function in post-stroke patients. NeuroRehabilitation 2018; 43(2):211–8.

34. Strong MJ, Donison NS, Volkening K. Alterations in tau metabolism in ALS and ALS-FTSD. Front Neurol 2020;11:598907.

35. Arai T, Hasegawa M, Akiyama H, et al. TDP-43 is a component of ubiquitin-positive tau-negative inclusions in frontotemporal lobar degeneration and amyotrophic lateral sclerosis. Biochem Biophys Res Commun 2006;351:602–11.

36. Lucia D, McCombe PA, Henderson RD, et al. Disorders of sleep and wakefulness in amyotrophic lateral sclerosis (ALS): a systematic review. Amyotroph Lateral Scler Frontotemporal Degener 2020; 16:1–9.

37. Ahmed RM, Newcombe REA, Piper AJ, et al. Sleep disorders and respiratory function in amyotrophic lateral sclerosis. Sleep Med Rev 2016;26:33–42.

38. Cykowski MD, Takei H, Schulz PE, et al. TDP-43 pathology in the basal forebrain and hypothalamus of patients with amyotrophic lateral sclerosis. Acta Neuropathol Commun 2014;2:171.

39. Sun X, Zhao X, Liu Q, et al. Study on sleep-wake disorders in patients with genetic and non-genetic amyotrophic lateral sclerosis. J Neurol Neurosurg Psychiatry 2020. jnnp-2020-324544.

40. Ferguson KA, Strong MJ, Ahmad D, et al. Sleep-disordered breathing in amyotrophic lateral sclerosis. Chest 1996;110:664–9.

41. Lo Coco D, Piccoli F, La Bella V. Restless legs syndrome in patients with amyotrophic lateral sclerosis. Mov Disord 2010;25:2658–61.

42. Puligheddu M, Congiu P, Arico D, et al. Isolated rapid eye movement sleep without atonia in amyotrophic lateral sclerosis. Sleep Med 2016;26:16–22.

43. Congiu P, Mariani S, Milioli G, et al. Sleep cardiac dysautonomia and EEG oscillations in amyotrophic lateral sclerosis. Sleep 2019;42(11):zsz164.

44. Malekshahi A, Chaudhary U, Jaramillo-Gonzalez A, et al. Sleep in the completely locked-in state (CLIS) in amyotrophic lateral sclerosis. Sleep 2019;42:42.

45. Soekadar SR, Born J, Birbaumer N, et al. Fragmentation of slow wave sleep after onset of complete locked-in state. J Clin Sleep Med 2013;9(9):951–3.

46. Boentert M. Sleep and sleep disruption in amyotrophic lateral sclerosis. Curr Neurol Neurosci Rep 2020;20(7):25.

47. Santos C, Braghiroli A, Mazzini L, et al. Sleep-related breathing disorders in amyotrophic lateral sclerosis. Monaldi Arch Chest Dis 2003;59(2): 160–5.

48. Barthlen GM, Lange DJ. Unexpectedly severe sleep and respiratory pathology in patients with amyotrophic lateral sclerosis. Eur J Neurol 2000; 7(3):299–302.

49. Vrijsen B, Buyse B, Belge C, et al. Noninvasive ventilation improves sleep in amyotrophic lateral sclerosis: a prospective polysomnographic study. J Clin Sleep Med 2015;11(5):559–66.

50. Crescimanno G, Sorano A, Greco F, et al. Heterogeneity of predictors of nocturnal hypoventilation in amyotrophic lateral sclerosis. Amyotroph Lateral Scler Frontotemporal Degener 2021;22: 46–52.

51. Muñoz-Lopetegi A, Graus F, Dalmau J, et al. Sleep disorders in autoimmune encephalitis. Lancet Neurol 2020;19(12):1010–22.

52. Sabater L, Gaig C, Gelpi E, et al. A novel non-rapid-eye movement and rapid-eye movement parasomnia with sleep breathing disorder associated with antibodies to IgLON5: a case series, characterisation of the antigen, and post-mortem study. Lancet Neurol 2014;13:575–86.

53. Gaig C, Iranzo A, Cajochen C, et al. Characterization of the sleep disorder of anti-IgLON5 disease. Sleep 2019;42:zsz133.

54. Bahtz R, Teegen B, Borowski K, et al. Autonatibodies against IgLON5: two new cases. J Neuroimmunol 2014;275:8.

55. Ramanan VK, Crum BA, McKeon A. Subacute encephalitis with recovery in IgLON5 autoimmunity. Neurol Neuroimmunol Neuroinflamm 2018;5:e485.

56. Gelpi E, Höftberger R, Graus F, et al. Neuropathological criteria of anti-IgLON5-related tauopathy. Acta Neuropathol 2016;132:531–43.

57. Iranzo A. Sleep and neurological autoimmune diseases. Neuropsychopharmacology 2020;45(1): 129–40.

58. Rao VR, Leguia MG, Tcheng TK, et al. Cues for seizure timing. Epilepsia 2020;62(Suppl1):S15–31.

59. Joo HR, Frank LM. The hippocampal sharp wave-ripple in memory retrieval for immediate use and consolidation. Nat Rev Neurosci 2018;19(12): 744–57.

60. Steriade M, Amzica F. Coalescence of sleep rhythms and their chronology in corticothalamic networks. Sleep Res Online 1998;1(1):1–10.

61. Vanhatalo S, Palva JM, Holmes MD, et al. Infraslow oscillations modulate excitability and interictal epileptic activity in the human cortex during sleep. Proc Natl Acad Sci U S A 2004;101(14):5053–7.

62. Parrino L, Vaudano AE. The resilient brain and the guardians of sleep: new perspectives on old assumptions. Sleep Med Rev 2018;39:98–107.

63. Halász P, Terzano MG, Parrino L. Spike-wave discharge and the microstructure of sleep-wake continuum in idiopathic generalized epilepsy. Neurophysiol Clin 2002;32(1):38–53.

64. Wang YQ, Zhang MQ, Li R, et al. The mutual interaction between sleep and epilepsy on the neurobiological basis and therapy. Curr Neuropharmacol 2018;16(1):5–16.

65. Evangelisti S, Testa C, Ferri L, et al. Brain functional connectivity in sleep-related hypermotor epilepsy. Neuroimage Clin 2017;17:873–81.

66. Weiss SA, Song I, Leng M, et al. Ripples have distinct spectral properties and phase-amplitude coupling with slow waves, but indistinct unit firing, in human epileptogenic hippocampus. Front Neurol 2020;11:174.

67. Terzano MG, Parrino L, Anelli S, et al. Effects of generalized interictal EEG discharges on sleep stability: assessment by means of cyclic alternating pattern. Epilepsia 1992;33(2):317–26.

68. Parrino L, Halasz P, Tassinari CA, et al. CAP, epilepsy and motor events during sleep: the unifying role of arousal. Sleep Med Rev 2006;10: 267–85.

69. Schomer DL, Lopez da Silva FH, editors. Niedermeyer's electroencephalography: basic principles, clinical applications, and related fields. 6th edition. Philadelphia: Lippincott Williams & Wilkins; 2011.

70. Çilliler AE, Güven B. Sleep quality and related clinical features in patients with epilepsy: a preliminary report. Epilepsy Behav 2020;102:106661.

71. Mutti C, Bernabè G, Barozzi N, et al. Commonalities and differences in NREM parasomnias and sleep-related epilepsy: is there a continuum between the two conditions? Front Neurol 2020;11: 600026.

72. Parrino L, De Paolis F, Milioli G, et al. Distinctive polysomnographic traits in nocturnal frontal lobe epilepsy. Epilepsia 2012;53:1178–84.

73. Halász P, Szűcs A. Sleep and epilepsy link by plasticity. Front Neurol 2020;11:911.

74. Samanta D, Al Khalili Y. Electrical status epilepticus in sleep. In: Dulebohn S, editor. StatPearls. Treasure Island (FL): StatPearls Publishing; 2020. p. 2–4.

75. Sánchez Fernández I, Takeoka M, Tas E, et al. Early thalamic lesions in patients with sleep-potentiated epileptiform activity. Neurology 2012;78(22): 1721–7.

76. Tassinari CA, Rubboli G. Cognition and paroxysmal EEG activities: from a single spike to electrical status epilepticus during sleep. Epilepsia 2006; 47(Suppl 2):40–3.

77. Hughes JR. A review of the relationships between Landau-Kleffner syndrome, electrical status epilepticus during sleep, and continuous spike-waves during sleep. Epilepsy Behav 2011;20(2):247–53.

78. Peng W, Ding J, Wang X. The managements and alternative therapies for comorbid sleep disorders in epilepsy. Curr Neuropharmacol 2020. https://doi.org/10.2174/1570159X19666201230142716.

79. Bisulli F, Vignatelli L, Naldi I, et al. Increased frequency of arousal parasomnias in families with nocturnal frontal lobe epilepsy: a common mechanism? Epilepsia 2010;51:1852–60.

80. Asioli GM, Rossi S, Bisulli F, et al. Therapy in sleep-related hypermotor epilepsy (SHE). Curr Treat Options Neurol 2020;22(1):1.

81. Puligheddu M, Melis M, Pillolla G, et al. Rationale for an adjunctive therapy with fenofibrate in pharmacoresistant nocturnal frontal lobe epilespy. Epilepsia 2017;58:1762–70.

82. Nobili L, Francione S, Mai R, et al. Surgical treatment of drug-resistant nocturnal frontal lobe epilepsy. Brain 2007;130(2):561–73.

83. Bergmann M, Prieschl M, Stefani A, et al. A prospective controlled study about sleep disorders in drug resistant epilepsy. Sleep Med 2020; 75:434–40.

84. Sun Y, Li J, Zhang X, et al. Case report: parasomnia overlap disorder induced by obstructive sleep hypopnea apnea syndrome: a case report and literature review. Front Neurosci 2020;14:578171.

85. Voysey ZJ, Barker RA, Lazar AS. The treatment of sleep dysfunction in neurodegenerative disorders. Neurotherapeutics 2020. https://doi.org/10.1007/s13311-020-00959-7.

86. Gehrman P, Gooneratne NS, Brewster GS, et al. Impact of Alzheimer disease patients' sleep disturbances on their caregivers. Geriatr Nurs (Minneap) 2018;39:60–5.

87. Pollak CP, Perlick D, Linsner JP, et al. Sleep problems in the community elderly as predictors of death and nursing home placement. J Community Health 1990;15:123–35.

88. Hope T, Keene J, Gedling K, et al. Predictors of institutionalization for people with dementia living at home with a carer. Int J Geriatr Psychiatry 1998; 13:682–90.

89. Mander BA, Marks SM, Vogel JW, et al. β-Amyloid disrupts human NREM slow waves and related hippocampus- dependent memory consolidation. Nat Neurosci 2015;18(7):1051–7.

90. Ferini-Strambi L, Hensley M, Salsone M. Decoding causal links between sleep apnea and Alzheimer's disease. J Alzheimers Dis 2021;80:29–40.

91. Shiota S, Takekawa H, Matsumoto SE, et al. Chronic intermittent hypoxia/reoxygenation facilitate amyloid-beta generation in mice. J Alzheimers Dis 2013;37: 325–33.

92. Liguori C, Mercuri NB, Nuccetelli M, et al. Obstructive sleep apnea may induce orexinergic system and cerebral β-amyloid metabolism dysregulation: is it a further proof for Alzheimer's disease risk? Sleep Med 2019;56:171–6.

93. Richards KC, Allen RP, Morrison J, et al. Nighttime agitation in persons with dementia as a manifestation of restless legs syndrome. J Am Med Dir Assoc 2020. S1525-8610(20)31012-4.

94. Borda MG, Jaramillo-Jimenez A, Oesterhus R, et al. Benzodiazepines and antidepressants: effects on cognitive and functional decline in Alzheimer's disease and Lewy body dementia. Int J Geriatr Psychiatry 2020. https://doi.org/10.1002/gps.5494.

95. St Louis EK, Boeve B. REM sleep behavior disorder: diagnosis, clinical implications, and future directions. Mayo Clin Proc 2017;92(11):1723–36.

96. Ferini-Strambi L, Galbiati A, Casoni F, et al. Therapy for insomnia and circadian rhythm disorder in Alzheimer disease. Curr Treat Options Neurol 2020;22(2):4.

97. AASM. International classification of sleep disorders. 3rd edition. Darien (IL): American Academy of Sleep Medicine; 2014.

98. Boeve BF. Pathophysiology of REM sleep behavior disorder and relevance to neurodegenerative disease. Brain 2007;130:2770–88.

99. De Cock VC, Vidailhet M, Leu S, et al. Restoration of normal motor control in Parkinson's disease during REM sleep. Brain 2007;30(Pt 2):450–6.

100. Plazzi G, Corsini R, Provini F, et al. REM sleep behavior disorders in multiple system atrophy. Neurology 1997;48(4):1094–7.

101. Melpignano A, Parrino L, Santamaria J, et al. Isolated rapid eye movement sleep behavior disorder and cyclic alternating pattern: is sleep microstructure a predictive parameter of neurodegeneration? Sleep 2019;42(10):zsz142.

102. Pham CK, Slowik JM. Rapid eye movement sleep behavior disorder. In: Dulebohn S, editor. StatPearls. Treasure Island (FL): StatPearls Publishing; 2020. p. 2–3.

103. Aurora RN, Zak RS, Maganti RK, et al. Best practice guide for the treatment of REM sleep behavior disorder (RBD) [published correction appears in. J Clin Sleep Med 2010;6(2):85–95.

104. Zuzuárregui JRP, During EH. Sleep issues in Parkinson's disease and their management. Neurotherapeutics 2020;17:1480–94.

105. Mantovani S, Smith SS, Gordon R, et al. An overview of sleep and circadian dysfunction in Parkinson's disease. J Sleep Res 2018;27(3):e12673.

106. Elfil M, Bahbah EI, Attia MM, et al. Impact of obstructive sleep apnea on cognitive and motor functions in Parkinson's disease. Mov Disord 2020;36:570–80.

107. Bargiotas P, Lachenmayer ML, Schreier DR, et al. Sleepiness and sleepiness perception in patients with Parkinson's disease: a clinical and electrophysiological study. Sleep 2019;42(4):zsz004.

108. Iliff JJ, Wang M, Liao Y, et al. A paravascular pathway facilitates CSF flow through the brain parenchyma and the clearance of interstitial solutes, including amyloid β. Sci Transl Med 2012;4(147): 147ra111.

109. Jessen NA, Munk AS, Lundgaard I, et al. The glymphatic system: a beginner's guide. Neurochem Res 2015;40(12):2583–99.

110. Piantino J, Lim MM, Newgard CD, et al. Linking traumatic brain injury, sleep disruption and post-traumatic headache: a potential role for glymphatic pathway dysfunction. Curr Pain Headache Rep 2019;23(9):62.

111. Xie L, Kang H, Xu Q, et al. Sleep drives metabolite clearance from the adult brain. Science 2013; 342(6156):373–7.

112. Wang J, Huang Q, Li N, et al. Triggers of migraine and tension-type headache in China: a clinic-based survey. Eur J Neurol 2013;20(4):689–96.

113. Barbanti P, Fabbrini G, Aurilia C, et al. A case-control study on excessive daytime sleepiness in episodic migraine. Cephalalgia 2007;27(10): 1115–9.

114. Boardman HF, Thomas E, Millson DS, et al. Psychological, sleep, lifestyle, and comorbid associations with headache. Headache 2005;45(6):657–69.

115. Dodick DW, Eross EJ, Parish JM, et al. Clinical, anatomical, and physiologic relationship between sleep and headache. Headache 2003;43(3): 282–92 [published correction appears in Headache 2004;44(4):384].

116. Lin YK, Lin GY, Lee JT, et al. Associations between sleep quality and migraine frequency: a cross-sectional case-control study. Medicine (Baltimore) 2016;95(17):e3554.

117. Rains JC. Sleep and migraine: assessment and treatment of comorbid sleep disorders. Headache 2018;58(7):1074–91.

118. Kelman L, Rains JC. Headache and sleep: examination of sleep patterns and complaints in a large clinical sample of migraineurs. Headache 2005; 45(7):904–10.

119. Lautenbacher S, Kundermann B, Krieg JC. Sleep deprivation and pain perception. Sleep Med Rev 2006;1 0(5):357–69.

120. Supornsilpchai W, Sanguanrangsirikul S, Maneesri S, et al. Serotonin depletion, cortical spreading depression, and trigeminal nociception. Headache 2006;46(1):34–9.

121. Headache Classification Committee of the International Headache Society (IHS) The International Classification of Headache Disorders, 3rd edition. Cephalalgia 2018;38(1):1–211.

122. Roccella M, Marotta R, Operto FF, et al. NREM sleep instability in pediatric migraine without aura. Front Neurol 2019;10:932.

123. Holland PR, Barloese M, Fahrenkrug J. PACAP in hypothalamic regulation of sleep and circadian rhythm: importance for headache. J Headache Pain 2018;19(1):20.

124. Teive HA, Kowacs PA, Maranhão Filho P, et al. Leao's cortical spreading depression: from experimental "artifact" to physiological principle. Neurology 2005;65(9):1455–9.

125. Schain AJ, Melo-Carrillo A, Strassman AM, et al. Cortical spreading depression closes paravascular space and impairs glymphatic flow: implications for migraine headache. J Neurosci 2017;37(11): 2904–15.

126. Aurora SK, Ahmad BK, Welch KMA, et al. Transcranial magnetic stimulation confirms hyperexcitability of occipital cortex in migraine. Neurology 1998;50: 1111–4.

127. Coppola G, Pierelli F, Schoenen J. Is the cerebral cortex hyperexcitable or hyperresponsive in migraine? Cephalalgia 2007;27(12):1427–39.

128. Phipps H, Mondello S, Wilson A, et al. Characteristics and impact of U.S. Military blast-related mild traumatic brain injury: a systematic review. Front Neurol 2020;11:559318.

129. Castriotta RJ, Wilde MC, Lai JM, et al. Prevalence and consequences of sleep disorders in traumatic brain injury. J Clin Sleep Med 2007;3(4):349–56.

130. Sommerauer M, Valko PO, Werth E, et al. Excessive sleep need following traumatic brain injury: a case-control study of 36 patients. J Sleep Res 2013; 22(6):634–9.

131. Modarres M, Kuzma NN, Kretzmer T, et al. EEG slow waves in traumatic brain injury: convergent findings in mouse and man. Neurobiol Sleep Circadian Rhythms 2016;1. S2451994416300025.

132. Parcell DL, Ponsford JL, Rajaratnam SM, et al. Self-reported changes to nighttime sleep after traumatic brain injury. Arch Phys Med Rehabil 2006; 87(2):278–85.

133. Wickwire EM, Williams SG, Roth T, et al. Sleep, sleep disorders, and mild traumatic brain injury. What we know and what we need to know: findings from a National Working Group. Neurotherapeutics 2016;13(2):403–17.

134. Aoun R, Rawal H, Attarian H, et al. Impact of traumatic brain injury on sleep: an overview. Nat Sci Sleep 2019;11:131–40.

135. Guo Z, Cupples LA, Kurz A, et al. Head injury and the risk of AD in the MIRAGE study. Neurology 2000;54(6):1316–23.

136. Iliff JJ, Chen MJ, Plog BA, et al. Impairment of glymphatic pathway function promotes tau pathology after traumatic brain injury. J Neurosci 2014; 34(49):16180–93.

137. Moretti L, Cristofori I, Weaver SM, et al. Cognitive decline in older adults with a history of traumatic brain injury. Lancet Neurol 2012;11(12):1103–11.

138. Smith DH, Johnson VE, Stewart W. Chronic neuropathologies of single and repetitive TBI: substrates of dementia? Nat Rev Neurol 2013;9(4):211–21.

Insomnia Burden and Future Perspectives

Samson G. Khachatryan, MD, PhD[a,b]

KEYWORDS

- Insomnia ● Social ● Burden ● Novel treatments ● Noninvasive stimulation therapy ● COVID-19
- Future perspectives

KEY POINTS

- Insomnia is a largely prevalent and impactful health condition.
- The social and economic burden of insomnia is high with direct and indirect costs far outweighing the burden of treatment.
- Acute insomnia remains an understudied entity yet waiting for establishing its role and therapeutic guidelines.
- Cognitive behavioral therapy for insomnia in the forms of direct or online delivery modalities is the firstline treatment option whenever available.
- Noninvasive stimulation therapy could further enhance the therapeutic options of insomnia.

INTRODUCTION

Insomnia is a prevalent symptom and disorder in the general population.[1] Insomnia comprises a list of disorders included in the International Classification of Sleep Disorders, third edition, (ICSD-3) unified under the frequently used term insomnia disorder. Insomnia may present in primary or secondary form; it is frequently divided into acute (short-term) and chronic insomnia disorders, which are defined as lasting not more than 3 months and more than 3 months, respectively.[2] According to prevalence studies, the prevalence of chronic insomnia varies from 6% to 15% in the general population, depending on age and other factors,[3,4] whereas the lifetime prevalence of short-term insomnia increases to 50%.[5,6] Insomnia is a cause for daytime symptoms, which are also necessary for fulfilling the diagnosis. These symptoms include lack of attention and concentration, memory problems, anxiety and mood swings, daytime sleepiness, somatic symptoms that lead to lack of productivity, absenteeism, and anxiety of unwanted workplace consequences. All the above-mentioned symptoms directly impact a person living in modern society. Insomnia is associated with serious distress, irrational thoughts, and bedtime rituals. Introduction and widespread use of personal devices in the twenty-first century has led to some behavioral changes in the population. Individuals frequently use smartphones and tablets in the evening and right before sleep. Social media development and increased online communication, and other engagements, if not self-controlled, lead to increased anxiety, often perceived before sleep. Sleep medicine is a well-known field for device-based therapeutic methods, and insomnia is also becoming such an entity. Although for decades pharmacologic and cognitive behavioral therapy for insomnia (CBT-I) were the mainstays of insomnia treatment, the term nonpharmacologic recently included some newer options, mostly noninvasive stimulation therapy (NIST).

Patients with insomnia together with the whole field of sleep medicine faced a recent challenge in the form of the coronavirus disease 2019 (COVID-19) pandemic, lockdowns, and serious changes in people's lives, work schedules, personal communications, and relationships. The

---

[a] Department of Neurology and Neurosurgery, National Institute of Health, Ministry of Health, Titogradyan 14, Yerevan 0087, Armenia; [b] Sleep and Movement Disorders Center, Somnus Neurology Clinic, Titogradyan 14, Yerevan 0087, Armenia
E-mail address: drsamkhach@gmail.com

Sleep Med Clin 16 (2021) 513–521
https://doi.org/10.1016/j.jsmc.2021.05.006
1556-407X/21/© 2021 Elsevier Inc. All rights reserved.

current state of different insomnia-related aspects will be discussed in this article, with an attempt to address possible future developments and research directions.

SOCIAL AND ECONOMIC BURDEN OF INSOMNIA

The social effects of insomnia are multidirectional and multilevel. Insomnia has implications for decreased productivity at work, absenteeism, and health care use with an estimated 29.1 million people affected in Europe.[7] In their study Bin and colleagues[8] aimed to understand the independent burden of insomnia on individual function and health care use. Controlling for a priori known confounders, such as female gender, older age, pain, and psychological distress, they found that insomnia was associated with higher odds of disability days, difficulties in daily activities, use of sleep medications, life dissatisfaction, and more frequent visits to general practitioners. The investigators reported that 1 in 20 subjects had significant insomnia associated with life dissatisfaction independent of other physical and psychiatric comorbidities and were frequent users of health care services.[8] Insomnia was associated with low levels of health-related quality of life (HRQOL),[9] and the latter was low even in those who were on sedative-hypnotic medications in a large database study from Japan. The investigators speculate that similar low HRQOL in treated and untreated insomniacs may express the overall low effect of treatment of insomnia, and also the possible specific impact their medications potentially have (dependency and residual effects).[10]

Economic implications are discouraging considering that insomnia causes a high economic burden through direct and indirect costs. The structure of direct costs mostly consists of health care consultations, transportation, prescription medication, over-the-counter products, and alcohol used as a sleep aid. Indirect costs include insomnia-related absenteeism and productivity losses.[11]

CLINICAL ASPECTS OF INSOMNIA
Acute Insomnia

Insomnia is not just one condition; it encompasses several disorders classified in ICSD-3: chronic insomnia disorder (CID) and short-term insomnia disorder (SID), along with other insomnia disorders.[2] There was a well-known shrinking approach performed in transition to ICSD-3, when several types of insomnia disorders, for example, psychophysiologic, paradoxic, idiopathic, and pediatric insomnia, were unified under one umbrella. A usual

clinical diagnostic consideration is to differentiate between acute and chronic insomnia. CID as a more disabling type with a greater impact on health and social aspects of life traditionally receives more attention. A big part of insomnia research is focused and goes on toward studying various aspects of CID. However, SID or acute insomnia (AI) is unique in being the first period in a patient's life when he or she experiences this condition. The clinician is facing a situation when there is no hint to future prognosis on whether this AI will progress into chronic insomnia or will limit within the time of SID (duration of less than 3 months). There is also a controversy on whether AI, which later developed into CID, was an independent condition or a debut of CID per se. Here we can go into analogy with the new daily persistent headache, which requires clinical monitoring to be later classified elsewhere.[12] However, AI is an important entity carrying some risks: (1) AI brings an unstable condition with patients being on the edge of falling into chronic insomnia if not approached adequately, (2) AI could be a debut of a psychiatric disorder, and (3) repetitive AI episodes without reaching the criteria of CID represent another underrated entity, which carries a big potential of preventing the transformation into chronic insomnia. Some questions that still need to be answered with more accuracy are presented in **Box 1**.

Some of these questions were addressed by researchers in the field. Perlis and colleagues[13] recently studied the proportion of AI cases that proceed to chronic insomnia versus those that are limited within 12 weeks. The investigators found the 1-year incidence rate for AI to be 27%. Surprisingly, within the AI population transition to chronic insomnia was not as high as one would expect (6.8%), and from initial good sleepers only 1.8% developed chronic insomnia on later assessments. Besides, there was a subpopulation of participants who were having bouts of AI without compliance with CID diagnostic criteria or recovery, repetitive AIs (persistent poor sleepers, 19.3%). Another 72.4% of participants with AI recovered their sleep.

AI is usually self-limited and does not need specific treatment.[14] However, in some cases, especially when prolonged but still within 3 months, it may require treatment. In such situations, the patients try different over-the-counter and mostly herbal drugs, and, when unsuccessful, decide to seek professional help. When prompted, physicians may consider "lighter" medications unsuccessful and offer pharmacologic therapy.[15] However, this issue is not systematically studied. In contrast to chronic insomnia, AI is a largely unclear entity in regard to treatment. The European Sleep Research Society's (ESRS) insomnia guideline declares no need to treat AI recommending to wait, as it will resolve with the elimination of stressor.[14] However, there are certain situations when patients demand rapid correction of their sleeplessness, and this is surprisingly an unexplored territory. If AI bears even some risk of transformation into CID, it deserves more attention in terms of systematic approach and guidelines; it could be a perfect home for prevention medicine.

Considering the leading role of CBT-I in the management of CID, it is a logical step to implement a brief modification of CBT-I. Studies are exploring the possibility of administering a "single-shot" of CBT-I to patients with AI in the general population and special populations. Ellis and colleagues[16] and Randall and colleagues[17] found that a single session of CBT-I was effective in the treatment of AI. However, there is still much to do to understand the effects and improve the management of AI.[18]

As the availability of CBT-I is always an issue even in developed countries, and in some, it may be even completely absent, the pharmacologic management of AI could be a frequent practice in many settings.[19] Yet, there is lack of research on this topic, and the available guidelines mostly do not cover AI management and are developed for chronic insomnia diagnosis and psychological, behavioral, and pharmacologic management.[14,20–22] Some other organizations developed their recommendations mostly for chronic insomnia.[23]

Insomnia phenotypes (subtypes) include usually, and this is generally accepted, sleep-onset, sleep-maintenance, and early morning awakening variants, and their combinations. This division is important both for the clinical understanding of insomnia and for the choice of therapeutic methods and prediction of the medication effect duration.

Nonpharmacologic Treatment of Chronic Insomnia

Both ESRS and American Academy of Sleep Medicine (AASM) insomnia guidelines recommend CBT-I as the first-line therapeutic option for chronic insomnia when available.[14,21] European insomnia guideline mentions CBT-I as a method with strong evidence without differentiating between main CBT-I components. The guideline was recently endorsed by the World Sleep Society gaining a larger geographic impact.[24] The newly updated AASM guideline on psychological and behavioral treatments for CID in adults, while reinforcing the leading role of CBT-I, also adds levels of strength to recommendations for different components and their combinations.[22] Multicomponent CBT-I is given the strongest recommendation, whereas stimulus control, sleep restriction, and relaxation therapies may also be used as a single-component therapy. Sleep hygiene is not recommended as a single-component therapy. The recent development of brief therapies for insomnia (BTI) led to having a deserved place within the recommendations, with multicomponent BTIs being recommended for CID. Strengthening the role of BTIs is a crucial step in making psychological and behavioral therapy for insomnia accessible and allowing wider population coverage. The clinicians are given freedom in choosing the best delivery modality for CBT-I; this is especially important for places where CBT-I is unavailable or for resource-poor countries.

Noninvasive Stimulation Therapies

NISTs are a group of device-based methods for the treatment of depression, anxiety, and other conditions. There are at least 4 modalities of NISTs studied in patients with insomnia: repetitive transcranial magnetic stimulation (rTMS), transcranial direct current stimulation (tDCS), transcranial alternating current stimulation (tACS), and transcutaneous vagus nerve stimulation (tVNS). The efficacy of rTMS in insomnia was systematically reviewed by Sun and colleagues,[25] who concluded that rTMS is an effective option for insomnia without serious side effects. Furthermore, tDCS is also a promising noninvasive location-specific technique with a potential to modulate total sleep time in healthy volunteers[26] and in patients with insomnia.[27] tDCS is further shown to be beneficial in improving sleep quality in patients with major depressive disorder.[28] Information on other NIST modalities (tACS and tVNS) is scarce and needs further research.[29,30]

Overall, the above-mentioned methods are not standardized; some are used more for research purposes, and it is hard to draw distant conclusions from the involved studies. However, as a potential therapeutic alternative or a combination option with CBT-I and sedative-hypnotic pharmacotherapy, these may be considered a promising and important direction for future development.

Pharmacologic Treatment of Chronic Insomnia

Although being a frequently used option in real-life practice the pharmacotherapy of insomnia remains within previously set limits. The two main guidelines on pharmacotherapy are published in recent years and encompass all the important evidence for medications in chronic insomnia.[14,21] However, the guidelines may differ in their recommendations for different drug classes. AASM's guideline presents differentiated recommendations regarding sleep-onset or sleep-maintenance insomnia phenotypes. Some important similarities and also differences exist between these 2 documents, which are summarized in **Table 1**. An important development of the recent decade is the introduction of the novel pharmacologic group of orexin receptor antagonists into medical practice. Suvorexant and other molecules of orexin system targeting drug class were able to show satisfactory results in the trials.[31] It means much to a field with nearly the same spectrum of pharmacologic options lasting for many years. The problems in insomnia pharmacotherapy include limited treatment duration, as most recommendations and guidelines restrict the drug use for around 1 month.

HEALTH CARE BURDEN OF INSOMNIA
Comorbid Insomnia

Being a frequent symptom or disorder encountered in different patient populations, insomnia is shown to be prevalent in medical, neurologic, and psychiatric disorders. Among medical disorders, where insomnia is a frequent comorbidity, patients with cardiovascular disorders are the largest group with high morbidity and mortality rates.[32] One would expect that showing insomnia as a risk or confounding factor for cardiovascular disorders raises its weight. In fact, for recent decades such reports were progressively accumulating.[33] Recent large-scale studies confirm that insomnia should be treated in a more focused way by respective specialist fields.

In a study of 1082 patients with coronary heart disease, insomnia was shown to be present in almost half of the participants (45%), and anxiety, female sex, and diabetes were the strongest risk factors for insomnia.[34]

Considering both insomnia and hypertension being bridged pathophysiologically through sympathetic overactivity, it is also probable that there could be an interrelation between these 2 conditions. In their meta-analysis, Li and colleagues[35] analyzed 14 prospective cohort studies involving 395,641 participants. Their results indicate that the presence of insomnia significantly increases the risk of hypertension. This and other similar findings strongly suggest that the role of insomnia should be made more important by analogy with sleep-disordered breathing's impact on cardiovascular risks.[35] Results from Sleep Heart Health Study involving around 5000 participants confirm the importance of objectively measured short sleep duration insomnia as a risk factor for incident cardiovascular disease.[36]

In another large cohort study of 487,200 adults conducted in China, Zheng and colleagues[33] were able to show that after a 10-year follow-up the insomnia symptoms among the participants were independent risk factors for overall cardiovascular incidence, especially in young adults and those without hypertension. The role of insomnia as a possible cardiovascular risk factor was indirectly seen from a study by Haaramo and colleagues,[37] who showed a link between insomnia symptoms and subsequent prescription of cardiovascular medications.

Insomnia in Neurologic Disorders

Insomnia is expectedly seen in many neurologic disorders. Among them, stroke, epilepsy, Parkinson disease (PD), and other central nervous system and peripheral nervous system disorders are associated with sleep disturbances and especially with insomnia.

Stroke has been linked to sleep and its disturbance for many years.[38,39] Although the central role for this relationship belongs to sleep-disordered breathing, other sleep disorders gain interest recently.[40] Similar to cardiovascular disorders, insomnia is also a frequent encounter in cerebrovascular disorders. A recent meta-analysis shows that insomnia is highly prevalent in all phases of stroke with prevalence for acute, subacute, and chronic phases being 40.7%, 42.6%, and 35.9%, respectively.[41] In their 6-year follow-up cohort study Li and colleagues[42] were able to establish the role of insomnia as a risk factor for increased mortality after first-ever stroke alongside old age, stroke recurrence in the first year of follow-up, and hypertension. Insomnia may also be a risk factor for stroke, as it was shown in a study of insomnia after traumatic brain injury.[43] Importantly, insomnia together with other sleep disorders may impact the functional recovery after stroke.[44]

Table 1
Comparison of AASM and ESRS guidelines for pharmacotherapy of chronic insomnia

Drugs AASM/ESRS	ESRS (2017)		AASM (2017)		
	Recommended	Level of Recommendation	Recommended	Level of Recommendation	Insomnia Phenotypes
Suvorexant	N/A	N/A	Yes	Weak	SMI
Eszopiclone	Yes	N/A	Yes	Weak	SOI, SMI
Zaleplon	Yes	N/A	Yes	Weak	SOI
Zolpidem	Yes	N/A	Yes	Weak	SOI, SMI
Triazolam	Yes	N/A	Yes	Weak	SOI
Temazepam	Yes	N/A	Yes	Weak	SOI, SMI
Ramelteon	No	Strong	Yes	Weak	SOI
Doxepin	Yes	Strong	Yes	Weak	SMI
Trazodone	Yes	Strong	No	Weak	N/A
Tiagabine	N/A	N/A	No	Weak	N/A
Diphenhydramine	Yes	Strong	No	Weak	N/A
Melatonin	No	Strong	No	Weak	N/A
Triptophan	N/A	N/A	No	Weak	N/A
Valerian	N/A	N/A	No	Weak	N/A

Abbreviations: AASM, American Academy of Sleep Medicine; ESRS, European Sleep Research Society; N/A, not available; SMI, sleep-maintenance insomnia; SOI, sleep-onset insomnia.

Epilepsy is a complex and prevalent neurologic disorder with special implications for mental health and HRQOL. Insomnia is a promising direction of study in epilepsy considering the strong effects of sleep deprivation and the relation of some epileptic syndromes to the state of sleep.[45] However, only in recent decades studies including or focused on insomnia and epilepsy interaction started to emerge.[46,47] In a study from our group insomnia disorder was nearly twice as high in patients with epilepsy compared with controls from the general population (46.2% vs 24.6%, $P<.05$).[48] Overall, the available studies indicate that insomnia is a prominent symptom or disorder in epilepsy (28.9%–51%), is more prevalent in epilepsy than in the general population, and is influencing the seizure frequency and HRQOL in patients with epilepsy.[49]

PD has strong connections to sleep disorders[50]; this is a bidirectional link with the central role given to rapid eye movement sleep behavior disorder, as a reliable predictor for the development of parkinsonism and strongly connected to synucleinopathies.[51] However, insomnia is also a prevalent complaint in this population having sometimes a multicomponent nature.[52] All insomnia phenotypes may be present—sleep-maintenance, sleep-onset, and early morning awakenings, although the first is more frequent and may stem from PD-associated factors.[50] Zhu and

colleagues[53] studied the factors associated with severity of insomnia in PD and found that depressive symptoms, motor fluctuations, and the use of higher doses of dopamine agonists may have impact.

Alzheimer disease (AD) is the most common type of neurodegenerative dementia.[54] Sleep is severely disturbed in AD and other dementias, especially in advanced stages, although this is mostly connected to circadian rhythm sleep disturbance well described in this group of patients.[55] Thinking about sleep disturbance and sleep deprivation as a risk factor for dementia and AD, in particular, has been a newer avenue of research for recent decade. The available data are scarce to choose specifically chronic insomnia as a separate risk factor for dementia. However, lack of sleep or disturbed sleep/sleep disorders were associated with a higher risk of cognitive decline and dementia in several studies.[56–58]

Overall, this is a promising new direction of dementia research, as finding a possible modifiable risk factor for dementia prevention will have an enormous positive impact on dementia practice and global health.

Insomnia in Psychiatric Disorders

Psychiatric patients report sleep issues on many occasions.[59] Insomnia has a high prevalence among hospitalized psychiatric patients. Especially patients with depression, psychotic disorder, and bipolar disorders report high rates of insomnia. Also, there is a tendency by psychiatrists to not treat insomnia as an independent clinical entity.[60] Chronic insomnia may pose a risk of developing psychiatric disorders especially when the patients are using sedative-hypnotic medications.[61] CBT-I may be efficacious also in some psychiatric disorders comorbid with insomnia.[62,63]

Drug-Induced Insomnia

Insomnia may be a consequence of medication used in common medical practice. These effects, however, are hard to be discriminated from primary insomnia or other secondary causes. Overall, regarding the drug effects on sleep, some controversial data exist. It is known that many commonly used cardiovascular and psychotropic drugs have the potential to influence sleep quality. There are a few studies or reviews on this topic.[64] A recent study by Doufas and colleagues[65] represents quite an extensive review of meta-analyses of randomized controlled trials of mostly psychotropic drugs and finds discrepancies between the results and leaflet information.

Insomnia at the Time of Pandemic and Lockdown

The recent COVID-19 pandemic introduced a new reality into people's lives. As the pandemic is still ongoing and there are serious concerns on how the virus will behave in the future, there should be a good understanding of how this will impact the population's and health workers' sleep.

There are 3 main effects of COVID-19 on sleep medicine: (1) sleep disturbances in response to home confinement and change of lifestyle, (2) sleep disorders due to COVID-19, (3) change of work schedules at the sleep centers.

Serious changes in the daily work and leisure schedules, and the introduction of distant learning, lack of natural light, psychological distress due to restrictions, and limitation of physical meetings are all influencing the mood and thoughts of people in different countries. Nearly any of the above-mentioned issues may be more or less connected to sleep disturbance. Indeed, some studies already investigated this aspect and found significant worsening of the pre-existing sleep disorders and de novo occurrence of insomnia and other sleep symptoms. In an online survey by Voitsidis and colleagues,[66] 37.6% of the 2427 respondents had insomnia. Other studies revealed similar findings, although with less prevalence of insomnia (19%).[67]

In a study by Mandelkorn and colleagues,[68] 58% of the responders reported dissatisfaction with their sleep. Importantly, sleeping pill consumption increased by 20%.

There is a chance in the future to have a more detailed image of the COVID-19-related sleep problems, and insomnia in particular, when the results of a collaborative multinational study effort will become available.[69] Sleep clinicians should be aware of what this situation brings to their potential patients to manage them adequately and tailor to the particular situations they are engaged with.

COVID-19 had brought serious workload increase also for health care providers who were and still are on the frontlines of this "war" against the greatest health challenge of modern times. In a meta-analysis of sleep disturbance prevalence among physicians and nurses, Salari and colleagues[70] found insomnia in 27.3% to 68.3% of physicians and 19.5% to 60% of nurses from included studies.

COVID-19 is manifested by a wide spectrum of various symptoms including neurologic and psychiatric expressions: anxiety, depression, anosmia, myalgia, epileptic seizures, and some others. In a meta-analysis by Deng and colleagues,[71] insomnia or poor sleep quality was found to be reported between 20.3% and 30.4% depending on the instrument used for assessment.

On the other hand, the situation with novel coronavirus infection became a big challenge for sleep medicine practice sites. The strict measures applied in the beginning were later substituted by a thoroughly controlled practice. The professional sleep societies responded well to the challenges, introducing position statements that instructed their members on how to organize the sleep medicine practice in the changed conditions. Nearly every step of sleep laboratory routine functioning was impacted by the COVID-19 situation. Diagnostic procedures (polysomnography, home sleep apnea testing, actigraphy) were limited, postponed, or temporarily discontinued. Positive airway pressure therapy was not possible to conduct as usual due to the risk of infection spread.[72–74]

The Dead End of Insomnia

Considering the overall burden insomnia has on one's health it is not surprising that in some patients the feeling of inevitable damage to their health would increase the psychological pressure and anxiety it brings. The pressure and anxiety may lead to further negative thinking, fear of bed, and avoidance of sleep. The patients would put more and more effort to improve their sleep and with every fail will recognize further their weakness in front of insomnia problem. Thus, discussing the negative effects of insomnia with patients needs a careful background assessment of their personality and expectations. Pushing excessively toward a wide spectrum of consequences, like the risk of dementia, cardiovascular disease, and so on, would play rather a down-bringing role in the whole therapeutic process. This issue should be addressed and have detailed recommendations to follow.

SUMMARY

There are certain areas where our understanding, management effectiveness, and targeted approach have great potential to improve. A better understanding of insomnia disorder and its mechanisms, types, and phenotypes will inevitably lead to a more targeted approach to each patient's needs. On the other hand, researchers continue to explore new therapeutic avenues. The introduction to the practice of a completely new drug class is one example of such a big step forward in enriching the armamentarium of anti-insomnia medications. Alternative nonpharmacologic treatment modalities will probably gain more evidence and will enter the list of recommended options for the treatment of insomnia.

CLINICS CARE POINTS

- Acute or short-term insomnia is a risk factor for chronic insomnia, and is still poorly investigated and lacks evidence-based guidelines.
- According to American and European guidelines the pharmacologic therapy of chronic insomnia should have limited duration.
- Nonpharmacologic treatment of chronic insomnia disorder in the form of cognitive-behavioral therapy for insomnia (CBT-I) is the most effective method and should be implemented if available.
- Noninvasive stimulation therapies are a promising new direction to help enhancing the practice of insomnia disorder in future.
- COVID-19 pandemic and lockdown caused increased occurrence of insomnia in general population, also among medical workers and infected patients.

REFERENCES

1. Kay-Stacey M, Attarian H. Advances in the management of chronic insomnia. BMJ 2016;354:i2123.

2. American Academy of Sleep Medicine. International classification of sleep disorders. 3rd edition. Darien, IL: American Academy of Sleep Medicine; 2014.

3. Ohayon M. Epidemiological study on insomnia in the general population. Sleep 1996;19(3 Suppl):S7–15.

4. Roth T. Insomnia: definition, prevalence, etiology, and consequences. J Clin Sleep Med 2007;3(5 Suppl):S7–10.

5. Breslau N, Roth T, Rosenthal L, et al. Sleep disturbance and psychiatric disorders: a longitudinal epidemiological study of young adults. Biol Psychiatry 1996;39(6):411–8.

6. Ancoli-Israel S, Roth T. Characteristics of insomnia in the United States: results of the 1991 national sleep foundation survey. I. Sleep 1999;22(Suppl 2): S347–53.

7. Wittchen HU, Jacobi F, Rehm J, et al. The size and burden of mental disorders and other disorders of the brain in Europe 2010. Eur Neuropsychopharmacol 2011;21(9):655–79.

8. Bin YS, Marshall NS, Glozier N. The burden of insomnia on individual function and healthcare consumption in Australia. Aust N Z J Public Health 2012; 36(5):462–8.

9. Kyle SD, Morgan K, Espie CA. Insomnia and health-related quality of life. Sleep Med Rev 2010;14(1): 69–82.

10. Mishima K, DiBonaventura Md, Gross H. The burden of insomnia in Japan. Nat Sci Sleep 2015;7:1–11.

11. Daley M, Morin CM, LeBlanc M, et al. The economic burden of insomnia: direct and indirect costs for individuals with insomnia syndrome, insomnia symptoms, and good sleepers. Sleep 2009;32(1): 55–64.

12. The international classification of headache disorders, 3rd edition (beta version). Cephalalgia 2013; 33(9):629–808.

13. Perlis ML, Vargas I, Ellis JG, et al. The Natural History of Insomnia: the incidence of acute insomnia and subsequent progression to chronic insomnia or recovery in good sleeper subjects. Sleep 2020; 43(6):zsz299.

14. Riemann D, Baglioni C, Bassetti C, et al. European guideline for the diagnosis and treatment of insomnia. J Sleep Res 2017;26(6):675–700.

15. Araújo T, Jarrin DC, Leanza Y, et al. Qualitative studies of insomnia: current state of knowledge in the field. Sleep Med Rev 2017;31:58–69.

16. Ellis JG, Cushing T, Germain A. Treating acute insomnia: a randomized controlled trial of a "single-shot" of cognitive behavioral therapy for insomnia. Sleep 2015;38(6):971–8.

17. Randall C, Nowakowski S, Ellis JG. Managing acute insomnia in prison: evaluation of a "one-shot" cognitive behavioral therapy for insomnia (CBT-I) intervention. Behav Sleep Med 2019;17(6):827–36.

18. Ellis JG. Cognitive behavioral therapy for insomnia and acute insomnia: considerations and controversies. Sleep Med Clin 2019;14(2):267–74.

19. Morin CM. Definition of acute insomnia: diagnostic and treatment implications. Sleep Med Rev 2012; 16(1):3–4.

20. Schutte-Rodin S, Broch L, Buysse D, et al. Clinical guideline for the evaluation and management of chronic insomnia in adults. J Clin Sleep Med 2008; 4(5):487–504.

21. Sateia MJ, Buysse DJ, Krystal AD, et al. Clinical practice guideline for the pharmacologic treatment of chronic insomnia in adults: an American Academy of Sleep Medicine clinical practice guideline. J Clin Sleep Med 2017;13(2):307–49.

22. Edinger JD, Arnedt JT, Bertisch SM, et al. Behavioral and psychological treatments for chronic insomnia disorder in adults: an American Academy of Sleep Medicine clinical practice guideline. J Clin Sleep Med 2021;17(2):255–62.

23. Qaseem A, Kansagara D, Forciea MA, et al. Management of chronic insomnia disorder in adults: a clinical practice guideline from the American College of Physicians. Ann Intern Med 2016;165(2): 125–33.

24. Members TF, Members GC, Morin CM, et al. Endorsement of European guideline for the diagnosis and treatment of insomnia by the world sleep society. Sleep Med 2021;81:124–6.

25. Sun N, He Y, Wang Z, et al. The effect of repetitive transcranial magnetic stimulation for insomnia: a systematic review and meta-analysis. Sleep Med 2020;77:226–37.

26. Frase L, Piosczyk H, Zittel S, et al. Modulation of total sleep time by transcranial direct current stimulation (tDCS). Neuropsychopharmacology 2016; 41(10):2577–86.

27. Frase L, Selhausen P, Krone L, et al. Differential effects of bifrontal tDCS on arousal and sleep duration in insomnia patients and healthy controls. Brain Stimul 2019;12(3):674–83.

28. Zhou Q, Yu C, Yu H, et al. The effects of repeated transcranial direct current stimulation on sleep quality and depression symptoms in patients with major depression and insomnia. Sleep Med 2020;70:17–26.

29. Wang HX, Wang L, Zhang WR, et al. Effect of transcranial alternating current stimulation for the treatment of chronic insomnia: a randomized, double-blind, parallel-group, placebo-controlled clinical trial. Psychother Psychosom 2020;89(1):38–47.

30. Jiao Y, Guo X, Luo M, et al. Effect of transcutaneous vagus nerve stimulation at auricular concha for insomnia: a randomized clinical trial. Evid Based Complement Alternat Med 2020;2020:6049891.

31. Kuriyama A, Tabata H. Suvorexant for the treatment of primary insomnia: a systematic review and meta-analysis. Sleep Med Rev 2017;35:1–7.

32. Cappuccio FP, Cooper D, D'Elia L, et al. Sleep duration predicts cardiovascular outcomes: a systematic review and meta-analysis of prospective studies. Eur Heart J 2011;32(12):1484–92.

33. Zheng B, Yu C, Lv J, et al. Insomnia symptoms and risk of cardiovascular diseases among 0.5 million adults: a 10-year cohort. Neurology 2019;93(23): e2110–20.

34. Frøjd LA, Munkhaugen J, Moum T, et al. Insomnia in patients with coronary heart disease: prevalence and correlates. J Clin Sleep Med 2021;17(5):931–8.

35. Li L, Gan Y, Zhou X, et al. Insomnia and the risk of hypertension: a meta-analysis of prospective cohort studies. Sleep Med Rev 2020;56:101403.

36. Bertisch SM, Pollock BD, Mittleman MA, et al. Insomnia with objective short sleep duration and risk of incident cardiovascular disease and all-cause mortality: sleep heart health study. Sleep 2018;41(6):zsy047.

37. Haaramo P, Rahkonen O, Hublin C, et al. Insomnia symptoms and subsequent cardiovascular medication: a register-linked follow-up study among middle-aged employees. J Sleep Res 2014;23(3):281–9.

38. Bassetti C, Aldrich M. Night time versus daytime transient ischaemic attack and ischaemic stroke: a prospective study of 110 patients. J Neurol Neurosurg Psychiatry 1999;67(4):463–7.

39. Hermann DM, Bassetti CL. Sleep apnea and other sleep-wake disorders in stroke. Curr Treat Options Neurol 2003;5(3):241–9.

40. Bassetti CLA, Randerath W, Vignatelli L, et al. EAN/ERS/ESO/ESRS statement on the impact of sleep disorders on risk and outcome of stroke. Eur J Neurol 2020;27(7):1117–36.

41. Hasan F, Gordon C, Wu D, et al. Dynamic prevalence of sleep disorders following stroke or transient Ischemic attack: systematic review and meta-analysis. Stroke 2021;52(2):655–63.

42. Li LJ, Yang Y, Guan BY, et al. Insomnia is associated with increased mortality in patients with first-ever stroke: a 6-year follow-up in a Chinese cohort study. Stroke Vasc Neurol 2018;3(4):197–202.

43. Ao KH, Ho CH, Wang CC, et al. The increased risk of stroke in early insomnia following traumatic brain injury: a population-based cohort study. Sleep Med 2017;37:187–92.

44. Fulk GD, Boyne P, Hauger M, et al. The impact of sleep disorders on functional recovery and participation following stroke: a systematic review and meta-analysis. Neurorehabil Neural Repair 2020; 34(11):1050–61.

45. Nobili L, de Weerd A, Rubboli G, et al. Standard procedures for the diagnostic pathway of sleep-related epilepsies and comorbid sleep disorders: an EAN, ESRS and ILAE-Europe consensus review. Eur J Neurol 2021;28(1):15–32.

46. Vendrame M, Yang B, Jackson S, et al. Insomnia and epilepsy: a questionnaire-based study. J Clin Sleep Med 2013;9(2):141–6.

47. Quigg M, Gharai S, Ruland J, et al. Insomnia in epilepsy is associated with continuing seizures and worse quality of life. Epilepsy Res 2016;122:91–6.

48. Khachatryan SG, Ghahramanyan L, Tavadyan Z, et al. Sleep-related movement disorders in a population of patients with epilepsy: prevalence and impact of restless legs syndrome and sleep bruxism. J Clin Sleep Med 2020;16(3):409–14.

49. Macêdo PJOM, Oliveira PS, Foldvary-Schaefer N, et al. Insomnia in people with epilepsy: a review of insomnia prevalence, risk factors and associations with epilepsy-related factors. Epilepsy Res 2017; 135:158–67.

50. Stefani A, Högl B. Sleep in Parkinson's disease. Neuropsychopharmacology 2020;45(1):121–8.

51. Fereshtehnejad SM, Montplaisir JY, Pelletier A, et al. Validation of the MDS research criteria for prodromal Parkinson's disease: longitudinal assessment in a REM sleep behavior disorder (RBD) cohort. Mov Disord 2017;32(6):865–73.

52. Wallace DM, Wohlgemuth WK, Trotti LM, et al. Practical evaluation and management of insomnia in Parkinson's disease: a review. Mov Disord Clin Pract 2020;7(3):250–66.

53. Zhu K, van Hilten JJ, Marinus J. The course of insomnia in Parkinson's disease. Parkinsonism Relat Disord 2016;33:51–7.

54. Bondi MW, Edmonds EC, Salmon DP. Alzheimer's disease: past, present, and future. J Int Neuropsychol Soc 2017;23(9–10):818–31.

55. Van Erum J, Van Dam D, De Deyn PP. Sleep and Alzheimer's disease: a pivotal role for the suprachiasmatic nucleus. Sleep Med Rev 2018;40:17–27.

56. Sindi S, Kåreholt I, Johansson L, et al. Sleep disturbances and dementia risk: a multicenter study. Alzheimers Dement 2018;14(10):1235–42.

57. Lu Y, Sugawara Y, Zhang S, et al. Changes in sleep duration and the risk of incident dementia in the elderly Japanese: the Ohsaki Cohort 2006 Study. Sleep 2018;41(10):zsy143.

58. Xu W, Tan CC, Zou JJ, et al. Sleep problems and risk of all-cause cognitive decline or dementia: an updated systematic review and meta-analysis. J Neurol Neurosurg Psychiatry 2020;91(3):236–44.

59. Szelenberger W, Soldatos C. Sleep disorders in psychiatric practice. World Psychiatry 2005;4(3):186–90.

60. Doghramji K, Tanielian M, Certa K, et al. Severity, prevalence, predictors, and rate of identification of insomnia symptoms in a sample of hospitalized psychiatric patients. J Nerv Ment Dis 2018;206(10): 765–9.

61. Chung KH, Li CY, Kuo SY, et al. Risk of psychiatric disorders in patients with chronic insomnia and sedative-hypnotic prescription: a nationwide population-based follow-up study. J Clin Sleep Med 2015;11(5):543–51.

62. Jansson-Fröjmark M, Norell-Clarke A. Cognitive behavioural therapy for insomnia in psychiatric disorders. Curr Sleep Med Rep 2016;2(4):233–40.

63. Raglan GB, Swanson LM, Arnedt JT. Cognitive behavioral therapy for insomnia in patients with medical and psychiatric comorbidities. Sleep Med Clin 2019;14(2):167–75.

64. Van Gastel A. Drug-induced insomnia and excessive sleepiness. Sleep Med Clin 2018;13(2):147–59.

65. Doufas AG, Panagiotou OA, Panousis P, et al. Insomnia from drug treatments: evidence from meta-analyses of randomized trials and concordance with prescribing information. Mayo Clin Proc 2017;92(1):72–87.

66. Voitsidis P, Gliatas I, Bairachtari V, et al. Insomnia during the COVID-19 pandemic in a Greek population. Psychiatry Res 2020;289:113076.

67. Kokou-Kpolou CK, Megalakaki O, Laimou D, et al. Insomnia during COVID-19 pandemic and lockdown: prevalence, severity, and associated risk factors in French population. Psychiatry Res 2020;290: 113128.

68. Mandelkorn U, Genzer S, Choshen-Hillel S, et al. Escalation of sleep disturbances amid the COVID-19 pandemic: a cross-sectional international study. J Clin Sleep Med 2021;17(1):45–53.

69. Partinen M, Bjorvatn B, Holzinger B, et al. Sleep and circadian problems during the coronavirus disease 2019 (COVID-19) pandemic: the International COVID-19 Sleep Study (ICOSS). J Sleep Res 2021;30(1):e13206.

70. Salari N, Khazaie H, Hosseinian-Far A, et al. The prevalence of sleep disturbances among physicians and nurses facing the COVID-19 patients: a systematic review and meta-analysis. Glob Health 2020; 16(1):92.

71. Deng J, Zhou F, Hou W, et al. The prevalence of depression, anxiety, and sleep disturbances in COVID-19 patients: a meta-analysis. Ann N Y Acad Sci 2020;1486(1):90–111.

72. Ramar K. AASM takes the pulse of the sleep field and responds to COVID-19. J Clin Sleep Med 2020;16(11):1939–42.

73. Altena E, Baglioni C, Espie CA, et al. Dealing with sleep problems during home confinement due to the COVID-19 outbreak: practical recommendations from a task force of the European CBT-I Academy. J Sleep Res 2020;29(4):e13052.

74. Gupta R, Kumar VM, Tripathi M, et al. Guidelines of the Indian Society for Sleep Research (ISSR) for Practice of Sleep Medicine during COVID-19. Sleep Vigil 2020;1–12. [Epub ahead of print].

Daylight Saving Time
Pros and Cons

Barbara Gnidovec Stražišar, MD, PhD[a,b,]*, Lea Stražišar[c]

KEYWORDS

- Daylight saving time • Standard time • Circadian system • Sleep • Social jet lag

KEY POINTS

- Daylight saving time is the practice of advancing clocks in the period of the year between spring and fall 1 hour ahead of standard time to adjust local time clock so that the peak of social activities coincide with daylight hours.
- Although the original rational for its implementation was to conserve energy, these effects are questionable or negligible.
- Daylight saving time transitions impact sleep with a cumulative effect on sleep deprivation and circadian misalignment with social jet lag potentially harming human health.
- Current status of scientific societies is that potential health consequences are greater with perennial daylight saving time.
- The subjects with highest risk for adverse health effects of daylight saving time are individuals with poor sleep quality and those with more extreme manifestations of chronotypes, more so people living on western edges of the time zones.
- Permanent standard time is most suitable for preventing dissociation between social and biologic clock and its potential harmful health effects.

INTRODUCTION

Daylight saving time (DST) is the practice of advancing clocks in the period of the year between spring and fall 1 hour ahead of standard time (ST). As a result, there is one 23-hour day in late winter or early spring and one 25-hour day in autumn, when the clocks are set back to return to ST. DST is a political issue that was adopted in most areas of Europe and North America and some parts of South America, southeastern Australia, and in New Zealand. In some countries DST is called the "summer time," because during warmer months of the year it allows extra daylight before darkness falls in the evening. DST therefore changes the local time, set by human societies, or the so-called "social clock," so that we start our social day (eg, work, school) 1 hour earlier to the sun clock.[1] The latter is set by the rotation of the Earth and shows the local time of the apparent progression of the sun. According to the sun clock, noon is the time period when the sun is highest and midnight being exactly halfway between dusk and dawn. Our daily rhythms are governed by the biologic circadian clock that follows the time of the sun clock.[2] The light of the sun and the darkness at night are the most potent zeitgebers that adjust the timing of our body clock and synchronize it with the sun clock. In modern society with living indoors and night illumination, however, social clock is rarely synchronized with sun or body clocks.[1]

The issue of DST is an indirect consequence of dividing the surface of Earth into time zones, which are theoretically centered around every 15th meridian.[3] We live according to the same clock time within a time zone. However, the social clocks report the actual sun time only at the locations

[a] Centre for Paediatric Sleep Medicine, Paediatric Department, General Hospital Celje, Celje, Slovenia; [b] Department of Clinical Medical Studies, College of Nursing in Celje, Celje, Slovenia; [c] CMS - Center for Sleep Disorders, Finžgarjeva 4, 1000 Ljubljana, Slovenia
* Corresponding author. Paediatric Department, General Hospital Celje, Oblakova 5, 3000 Celje, Slovenia.
E-mail address: Barbara.gnidovec-strazisar@sb-celje.si

Sleep Med Clin 16 (2021) 523–531
https://doi.org/10.1016/j.jsmc.2021.05.007

directly on an hour-meridian. For practical purposes time zones are often much wider than to span only one sun-hour, increasing the discrepancy between the sun clock and the social clock inside the individual time zone. DST with assigning the respective location to one time zone further east, additionally disrupts these relationships. The actual increase of the discrepancy between the social and the sun clocks is even larger than just 1 hour because of different resynchronization dynamics.[4] This increases the gap between the social and biologic clocks and potentially harms human health.[2]

HISTORY OF DAYLIGHT SAVING TIME

The modern concept of DST was introduced in 1895 by George Vernon Hudson, an entomologist from New Zealand.[5] He proposed a 2-hour time shift so he would have more after-work hours of sunshine to go bug hunting in the summer. However, the earliest known reference to DST is tracked back to 1784, when Benjamin Franklin, at that time American minister to France, discussed a waste of candles because of the extended nightlife in Paris in a letter to the editor of *Journal de Paris*.[6] He suggested Parisians could economize candle usage and decrease energy expenditure simply by earlier rising in the morning, therefore changing the hour of their activity to make the best use of the daytime sunshine.

Similar observation was made more than 100 years later by William Willet, an English designer and builder of stately houses with special interest in light.[6] He realized "the waste of daylight" and proposed shifting the clock forward between April and September to save the daylight. This would allow some of the early morning's wasted sunlight to be used in the evening, and yet would not change anyone's normal waking time.[6] He recalculated the overall financial benefits of his proposed scheme reducing the ordinary expenditure on electric light, gas, oil, and candles. Additional benefit would be in the longevity of coal supplies because less coal would be required for the production of gas and electric lighting. Willet also argued that the extra hours spent outdoors, instead in the condition of the artificial light, would have beneficial effects on improvement of overall health. If exposed to more sunshine, people would suffer less from rickets, anemia, and eyestrain. He anticipated that daylight later in the evening might shorten sleep; however, for those with late chronotype, he suggested they would actually sleep better because more light in waking hours would leave more darkness for sleeping hours.[6]

Willet's idea of DST was not accepted at that time because of potential undue public inconvenience and interference with the ordinary measurement of time. However, with the beginning of World War I the energy savings once again came into play and whereas the British Parliament discussed the DST idea year after year, the Germans decided to implement it in 1916 to minimize the use of artificial lighting and save fuel for the war effort.[6] The decision was soon followed globally, and DST was implemented in most European countries, the United States, Russia, and many other countries. Most of them reverted back to ST after World War I and reinstalled DST in World War II only for it to be dismissed shortly thereafter.[6] Many countries have used it at various times since then, and particularly since the 1970s energy crisis DST was widely adopted because of the perception that it could save energy. Today DST is observed in nearly 80 countries, including the European Union (EU), the United States, Canada, and parts of Australia and in New Zealand. Most countries experiencing DST are within the higher latitude areas, where the use of DST minimizes exposure to seasonal variation in the availability of natural daylight.[7]

DAYLIGHT SAVING TIME PROS
Daylight Saving Time and Energy Saving

The original rationale for DST implementation was to conserve energy and interestingly, some have even named it as "daytime savings time." There is, however, little evidence in the current literature to support that DST policy actually saves energy. Although some studies have shown minimal decrease in electricity demands,[8] others on the contrary showed increased consumption mainly on account of increasing electricity expenditure for heating and cooling.[9] In a meta-analysis of the various studies on energy savings from DST, Havranek and colleagues[10] reported the mean estimate of 0% to 34% savings of total energy consumption during the days when DST was applied. Energy savings were larger for countries farther away from the equator, whereas subtropical regions consumed more energy because of DST.

These energy studies rarely compared data for longer periods of DST implementation with electricity consumption data from non-DST periods. Many of the studies were also limited to electrical demands only in residential sectors. Thus, in a natural experiment data set where DST had been observed for several years before it was stopped, Choi and colleagues[11] analyzed the effect of DST by direct comparison of the electricity demands in the period of DST adoption and the period of non-DST regime. Overall, they did not find any DST effect on electricity demand; however, the results showed strong redistribution effect by reducing electricity demands substantially in the late afternoon and early evening, thus supporting the use of DST as a way to reduce peak electricity demand.[8]

Other Possible Benefits of Daylight Saving Time

The aforementioned studies on energy conservation show the effects of DST on energy consumption are too small to justify the biannual time-shifting. Other aspects of DST that might prove more important could be increased opportunity for leisure and physical activity during summer months with their potential impact on enhanced public health, but these are often difficult to estimate. Moreover, the limited research of DST effect on physical activity showed no impact on moderate to vigorous physical activity[12] or only a change in physical activity pattern with unknown impact on overall physical activity levels.[13]

Other arguments in favor of DST could be increased safety and economic growth. Although Doleac and Sanders[14] indeed showed lower criminal rate following the shift to DST, there is less conclusive evidence for economic benefits. Calandrillo and Buehler[15] in their economic analysis suggested the advantages of DST would significantly outweigh the potential costs of DST during winter months. In contrast, Kamstra and colleagues[16] described markedly lower equity return in international markets on DST weekends. This "daylight saving anomaly" in financial markets was thought to be consistent with desynchronizing research that has identified the effect of changes in sleep patterns on judgment, anxiety, reaction time, problem solving, and accidents.[4]

DAYLIGHT SAVING TIME CONS
Daylight Saving Time, Sleep, and Circadian System

DST causes twice-yearly adjustment of local time clock so that the peak of social activities coincides with daylight hours. Contrary to general public belief, these adjustments to 1-hour time change do not occur immediately and without consequences. In has long been appreciated that DST transitions impact sleep by disrupting sleep duration, quality, and placement.[17] DST-induced misalignment between social and biologic circadian clock may persist for about 1 week after the transition, or possibly even longer,[18] with its main impact on sleep continuity and sleep efficiency.[19]

Direct sleep measurements have shown that circadian sleep advance, imposed by transition to DST in spring, was associated with increased sleep latency and up to 1 hour shorter sleep in the first week after the transition.[20,21] The cumulative sleep loss was even greater in adolescents and young adults.[22] At the same time sleep was more fragmented,[23] resulting in lower sleep efficiency and contributing to the overall sleep deprivation. However, there is little evidence of extra sleep because of greater sleep opportunity on the autumn shift back to ST. The resilience of pre-transition bedtimes resulted in significantly earlier rise times with the net loss of sleep across the first week after autumn transition.[17] Sleep-onset latency, sleep efficiency, and wake during sleep onset were also disrupted.[23,24]

The effect of DST transitions on sleep is greatly influenced by the chronotype and prior habitual sleep duration. Habitual long sleepers were shown to adjust more easily to the imposed clock change and the detrimental effects of the introduction of DST were significantly more pronounced for people with previous sleep debt.[25] Lahti and colleagues[25] suggested that morning types of chronotype would have less problems in adjusting to DST transition in spring. Similarly, Schneider and Randler,[26] studying daytime sleepiness in adolescents on spring transition to DST, revealed evening types to be sleepier than morning types after the transition even when controlling for individual differences in baseline sleepiness, thus confirming the assumption of relative ease of DST adjustment in morning types. Maintenance of sleep homeostasis after 1-hour time loss can therefore be particularly difficult for adolescents and young adults because of their physiologic sleep phase delay.[22]

Extreme circadian preference is likely to influence the duration of the adjustment. Sleep timing is subject to seasonal change and is influenced to a great extent by morning light, specifically sunrise times.[27] The influence is greatest at higher latitudes where there are large seasonal differences in the daily photoperiod.[28,29] The practice of yearly forward and backward transition of social clock reduces the ability of human biologic clock to seasonal adjustment with sleep placement being resistant to the socially imposed clock time throughout DST.[30] Therefore, adjustment of timing of sleep and activity to external clock time remained incomplete, even after 4 weeks, which was particularly the case for late chronotypes.[18] Following the autumn transition adjustment of sleep was complete in 1 to 2 weeks.[30]

In modern environments with greater availability of electrical lightning, sleep timing and duration seem to be more strongly associated with actual light exposure, including natural and electrical light, than merely the sun time.[31] This is especially the case in adolescents, because of higher sensitivity of their circadian system to light signals.[32] DST prioritizes the availability of evening daylight at the cost of morning daylight. Therefore, in a combination with urban lifestyle with artificial light at night and lack of daylight because of more time spent indoors, a reduction of the morning light because of DST leads to more difficulties to keep biologic clocks entrained with the advanced social time and to maintain vigilance and good work/school performance in morning hours.[33]

DST-induced circadian misalignment is also dependent on the geographic position inside the time zone, being more prevalent at locations further west, because difference between the social clock and the body clock increases toward the western edges of time zones.[3] It has been shown that in western edges of time zones average sleep duration is up to 19 minutes shorter than in eastern edges.[34] Therefore, DST-induced effects on the circadian system are more severe and harder to recover from in western than in eastern regions of a given time zone.[35] Recently, a large-scale sociodemographic survey in Czech Republic confirmed significant correlation of chronotype with latitude and longitude even in a small geographic area with later chronotype being more prevalent in western parts, increasing further the vulnerability of the late chronotypes, especially adolescents and people living alone without a partner.[33]

Emerging evidence suggests certain individuals are more vulnerable to twice-yearly phase shifts because of DST. The effect of DST transitions on sleep continuity are likely to be more pronounced in individuals with poor sleep quality and those with more extreme manifestations of chronotypes, more so in people living on western edges of the time zones.[19] Besides adolescents, young adults and other late chronotypes, even children and those with a morning-type preference, such as elderly, might be vulnerable to likely more disrupting effect of the light in the evenings following the spring clock change.[19] It is also possible that children and adolescents whose brains are still developing are more susceptible to the adverse health effects that occur following the DST transition.[36]

These different negative outcomes associated with DST transition may be associated with disruptions in the underlying genetic mechanisms that contribute to the expression of the circadian clock and its behavioral manifestation, such as chronotype.[37] Sleep time shifts cause global disruption in peripheral gene expression, and even the short-time sleep deprivation that occurs following the transition to DST may alter epigenetic and transcriptional profile of core circadian clock genes.[38]

Daylight Saving Time and Health

Scientific studies highlighted the detrimental effect of DST on sleep continuity in both transition periods with its cumulative effect on sleep deprivation. Sleep deprivation, however, is known to have many adverse health effects. Probably the most studied is the possible effect of DST-induced sleep deprivation in connection with cardiovascular health. Several clinical studies reported that transitions to DST increase the risk of cardiovascular and cerebrovascular problems, bringing significant excess mortality for all circulatory deaths,[39] and total mortality rates.[40,41] Even modest sleep deprivation and circadian misalignment may influence increased cardiovascular risks with increase in sympathetic tone and catecholamine levels,[42,43] lower vagal tone, resulting in increased heart rate and blood pressure,[44] and a release of proinflammatory cytokines.[45,46] The same mechanisms are known to provoke atrial fibrillation. Recently, Chudow and colleagues[47] found significant increase in mean atrial fibrillation admissions over the first days and entire week following the DST springtime transition compared with the yearly mean. This increase, however, persisted only in women and no significant differences in atrial fibrillation rate were found following the autumn transition back to ST.

Circadian rhythm disruption has been associated also with increased risk of ischemic stroke. Stroke onset shows a pattern of diurnal variation, with a peak in morning hours.[48] DST not only shifts the pattern of diurnal variation in stoke onset[49] but in the first 2 days after DST transition also increases their rate.[50] The effect is, however, diluted when observing the whole week after transition. As for atrial fibrillation, women were more susceptible than men, and other risk factors were advanced age and malignancy.[50]

Other prominent DST-associated elevated health risk clusters besides cardiovascular and cerebrovascular diseases include injuries, mental and behavioral disorders, and immune-related diseases.[51] Barnes and Wagner[52] showed shorter sleep on Mondays directly following the switch to DST mediated more workplace injuries with greater severity. However, best studied injury rates in relation to DST are the possible injuries from road traffic collisions and pedestrian injuries. The first systematic review of the literature, relating to the impact of DST on road safety showed inconsistent results from the studies of short-term impact of DST transition on road traffic collisions.[53] Of 16 eligible studies for the transition into DST, most (44%) showed no change in collisions. Only six studies reported an increase in collision rate that was largely attributed to sleep disruption. Similar results were obtained for the autumn shift, regardless of the improved lighting in the morning with its reduction in the evening, when the collision risk was supposed to be higher. Fifteen studies that provided relevant data showed exactly the same proportion of studies that reported a decrease, an increase, or no change in collision rate. These studies may, however, be biased, because they commonly compared collision rates after DST start with those in the preceding week or two. Robb and Barnes[54] argued that observed decrease in falls and home or community injuries before DST transition in their study is accounted for by behavioral change anticipating DST introduction. They suggested such "anticipation effect" may also be responsible for negative findings about DST influence on traffic accidents. Similarly, the aforementioned studies did not evaluate the collision risk in chronobiologic context, quantifying DST, time of day, and time zone effect. By doing so, Fritz and colleagues,[35] using large US registry data of more than 730,000 motor vehicle accidents, observed that spring DST significantly increased fatal motor vehicle accident risk by 6% in the week after DST transition compared with the risk of any other week of the year. Effects were more pronounced in the morning and in locations further west within the time zone, probably because of higher levels of circadian misalignment.

In contrast, the long-term impact findings suggested a positive effect of DST with reduction in collisions, injuries, and fatalities.[53] The reported beneficial effects of DST on road safety were most pronounced for pedestrians and cyclists,[55] with greater collision risk posed to pedestrians following the autumn shift from DST to ST.[56] However, the overall magnitude of these effects tended to be small.[53] Additionally, such a stringent causal conclusion is questionable because in several weeks observation period there might be significant changes in many other risk factors, such as traffic flow, weather conditions, photoperiod, and associated behavioral characteristics that were not controlled for. Therefore, it seems that beneficial long-term effects are more attributable to seasonal change rather than DST per se.[35]

DST transitions interfere with the timing of daylight, and in addition to disturbance of sleep lead also to the disturbance of circadian rhythms.[30] The latter has been implicated in the cause of mood disorders.[57] However, once again the results of different studies on DST association with different mental and behavioral disorders gave mixed results. Although some studies have shown that the transition from DST to ST in autumn is indeed associated with an increase in the incidence rate of unipolar depressive episodes[58] and suicide,[40,59] others found no association of the transition with hospital admissions for mood disorders.[60–62] Most of the mentioned studies only compared incidence of mood disorders shortly before and after the DST transitions. In a direct comparison of sleep timing and winter pattern of mood seasonality in Russian children and adolescents, evaluated in a steadier state of prolonged periods of permanent DST and permanent ST, Borisenkov and colleagues[63] observed 2% to 3% increase in the rate of symptoms of winter depression. Furthermore, in the group of adolescents from 10 to 17 years they found also a prominent dissociation between social and biologic clocks, the so-called "social jet lag."[2] Social jet lag is widespread among residents of industrialized countries and it is well known to be associated with obesity[64,65] and metabolic syndrome,[66] and is therefore one of many factors contributing to the epidemic of overweight and obesity that is of great concern especially in children and adolescents. Discrepancy between biologic and social timing, imposed by DST, has been shown to be associated also with poor academic performance,[67–70] cardiometabolic risk,[71] and depression.[72]

DAYLIGHT SAVING TIME CONSENSUS STATEMENTS

In light of the current evidence, the European Commission in autumn 2018 decided that biannual clock change in Europe would be abolished. The European Parliament voted to end mandatory DST by the 2021.[73] There is, however, an ongoing debate whether Europe as a whole should choose perennial ST or DST. Scientific associations mostly agreed that indirect evidence suggests that the risk of negative effects on public health and safety of perennial DST are higher than under perennial ST.[74] Society for Research on Biological Rhythms engaged experts in the field, who took the position that, based on comparisons of large populations living in DST or ST or on western versus eastern edges of time zones, the advantages of permanent ST outweighed switching to DST annually or permanently.[1] European Biological Rhythms Society, European Sleep Research Society, and Society for Research on Biological Rhythms published a joint statement declaring that permanent ST is the best option for public health.[75] The same position was taken also by 36 of 37 European national sleep societies joined in the Assembly of National Sleep Societies at their annual delegates meeting in St. Petersburg, Russia in May 2019 (personal communication). Recently, American Academy of Sleep Medicine similarly published a position statement that the United States should eliminate seasonal time change in favor of a national, fixed, year-round time.[76] By their position current evidence best supports the adoption of year-round ST, which aligns best with human circadian biology and has the potential to produce benefits for public health and safety.[76]

Although most of the scientific community believes permanent ST is the best option for public health, public preference might not be the same. In an EU study that included less than 1% of the EU population, 84% of respondents voted to abolish clock change.[77] However, more than half of the participants would keep perennial DST. Although most of the respondents as the main argument in favor of perennial ST mentioned general health considerations, the main argument for perennial DST respondents was evening leisure time activities, which are facilitated by the prolonged availability of daylight. Increased quality of life with prioritizing social relationship and leisure time activities is a protective factor against many health-related problems, including cognitive decline and dementia.[78] However, self-reported satisfaction scores in association with DST were found to be negatively associated with individual well-being.[79] The switch to permanent DST would negate beneficial effects of delaying school start times on adolescents' sleep habits, mood, and behavior.[80] Additionally, the results of the EU survey[77] are caused by the small sample and bias (70% of the participants were German), far from representative and hardly reflecting public preference.[74]

SUMMARY

There is substantial evidence that DST transitions have a cumulative effect on sleep deprivation with its adverse health effects. However, potential benefits, especially in regard to energy saving, are questionable or negligible. DST-induced manipulations with social clock may lead to prolonged disturbances of human circadian system. The circadian misalignment between social and biologic clocks (ie, social jet lag) is potentially harmful to human health. The European Commission therefore decided that biannual clock change in Europe would be abolished by 2021.[73] However, the COVID-19 pandemic postponed this decision

before reaching the final agreement on choosing perennial ST over perennial DST. Thus, this March EU once again switched their clocks to DST and it is hoped in autumn it will change back to ST for the last time. The current status of scientific societies is that potential health consequences would be greater with yearlong DST. There is a minority of people in the population who would not have a problem with perennial DST. The specific subjects with highest risk are individuals with poor sleep quality and those with more extreme manifestations of chronotypes, more so people living on western edges of the time zones. Permanent ST would therefore be most suitable for preventing dissociation between social and biologic clock and its potential harmful health effects.

CLINICS CARE POINTS

- Before spring transition to DST have a good and sufficient sleep, because the detrimental effects of the introduction of DST are significantly more pronounced for people with previous sleep debt.

- DST prioritizes the availability of evening daylight at the cost of morning daylight. Therefore, on transition to DST try to increase exposure to the light in the morning to keep the biologic clock entrained with the advanced social time and to maintain vigilance and good work/school performance in morning hours.

- Take special care at work on Mondays directly following the switch to DST because shorter sleep caused by the transition mediated more workplace injuries with greater severity.

- In the first week after DST transition take special care in road traffic, especially in the morning because spring DST shift significantly increased fatal motor vehicle accidents risk.

- The European Commission decided to abolish biannual clock change. In light of the current indirect evidence advocate for perennial ST adoption, which aligns best with human circadian system and has the potential to produce benefits for public health and safety.

DISCLOSURE

Barbara Gnidovec Stražišar discloses lecture fees from Medis d.d. that are not relevant for the article. Lea Stražišar has nothing to disclose.

REFERENCES

1. Roenneberg T, Wirz-Justice A, Skene DJ, et al. Why should we abolish daylight saving time? J Biol Rhythms 2019;34:227–30.
2. Roenneberg T, Merrow M. The circadian clock and human health. Curr Biol 2016;26:R432–43.
3. Roenneberg T, Winnebeck EC, Klerman EB. Daylight saving time and artificial time zones: a battle between biological and social times. Front Psycol 2019;10:944.
4. Meira e Cruz M, Miyazawa M, Manfredini R, et al. Impact of daylight saving time on circadian timing system: an expert statement. Eur J Intern Med 2019;60:1–3.
5. Obituary. George Vernon Hudson, F.R.S.N.Z. (1867-1946). Trans Proc R Soc New Zealand 1946;76:264.
6. Prerau D. Seize the daylight: the curious and contentious story of daylight saving time. New York: Thunder's Mouth Press; 2005. p. 1–276.
7. Martin-Olalla JM. The long term impact of daylight saving time regulations in daily life at several circles of latitude. Sci Rep 2019;9:18466.
8. Mirza FM, Bergland O. The impact of daylight saving time on electricity consumption: evidence from southern Norway and Sweden. Energy Policy 2011;39:3558–71.
9. Kotchen MJ, Grant LE. Does daylight saving time save energy? Evidence from a natural experiment in Indiana. Rev Econ Stat 2011;93:1172–85.
10. Havranek T, Herman D, Irsova Z. Does daylight saving save energy? A meta-analysis. Energy J 2018;39:35–61.
11. Choi S, Pellen A, Masson V. How does daylight saving time affect electricity demands? An answer using aggregate data from a natural experiment in Western Australia. Energy Econ 2017;66:247–60.
12. Zick CD. Does daylight saving time encourage physical activity? J Phys Activity Health 2014;11:1057–60.
13. Rosenberg M, Wood L. The power of policy to influence behaviour change: daylight saving and its effect on physical activity. Aust NZ J Public Health 2010;34:83–8.
14. Doleac JL, Sanders NJ. Under the cover of darkness: how ambient light influences criminal activity. Rev Econ Stat 2015;97:1093–103.
15. Calandrillo SP, Buehler DE. Time well spent: an economic analysis of daylight saving time legislation. Wake Forest Law Rev 2008;43:45–91.
16. Kamstra MJ, Kramer LA, Levi MD. Losing sleep at the market: the daylight saving anomaly. Am Econ Rev 2000;90(4):1005–11.
17. Monk TH, Folkard S. Adjusting to changes to and from daylight saving time. Nature 1976;261:688–9.
18. Hadlow NC, Brown S, Wardrop R, et al. The effects of season, daylight saving and time of sunrise on serum cortisol in a large population. Chronobiol Int 2014;31:243–51.
19. Harrison Y. The impact of daylight saving time on sleep and related behaviours. Sleep Med Rev 2013;17:285–92.
20. Lahti TA, Leppämäki S, Lönnqvist J, et al. Transition to daylight saving time reduces sleep duration plus sleep efficiency of the deprived sleep. Neurosci Lett 2006;406:174–7.
21. Sexton AL, Beatty TKM. Behavioral responses to daylight saving time. J Econ Behav Organ 2014;107:290–307.
22. Medina D, Ebben M, Milrad S, et al. Adverse effects of daylight saving time on adolescents' sleep and vigilance. J Clin Sleep Med 2015;11:879–84.
23. Lahti TA, Leppämäki S, Lönnqvist J, et al. Transition into and out of daylight saving time compromise sleep and the rest-activity cycles. BMC Physiol 2008;8. Article 3.
24. Harrison Y. Individual response to the end of daylight saving time is largely dependant on habitual sleep duration. Biol Rhythm Res 2013;44:319–401.
25. Lahti TA, Leppämäki S, Ojanen S-M, et al. Transition into daylight saving time influences the fragmentation of the rest-activity cycle. J Circadian Rhythms 2006;4:1.
26. Schneider A-M, Randler C. Daytime sleepiness during transition into daylight saving time in adolescents: are owls at higher risk? Sleep Med 2009;10:1047–50.
27. Roenneberg T, Kumar CJ, Merrow M. The human circadian clock entrains to sun time. Curr Biol 2007;17:R44–5.
28. Friborg O, Rosenvinge JH, Wynn R, et al. Sleep timing, chronotype, mood, and behaviour at an arctic latitude (69°). Sleep Med 2014;15:798–807.
29. Lowden A, Lemos N, Gonçalves M, et al. Delayed sleep in winter related to natural daylight exposure among arctic day workers. Clocks Sleep 2018;1:105–16.
30. Kanterman T, Juda M, Merrow M, et al. The human circadian clock's seasonal adjustment is disrupted by daylight saving time. Curr Biol 2007;17:1996–2000.
31. Shochat T, Santhi N, Herer P, et al. Sleep timing in late autumn and late spring associates with light exposure rather than sun time in college students. Front Neurosci 2019;13:882.
32. Crowley SJ, Cain SW, Burns AC, et al. Increased sensitivity of the circadian system to light in early/mid-puberty. J Clin Endocrinol Metab 2015;100:4067–73.
33. Sládek M, Kudrnáčová R, Adámková V, et al. Chronotype assessment via a large scale socio-demographic survey favours yearlong standard

time over daylight saving time in central Europe. Sci Rep 2020;10:1419.

34. Guintella O, Mazzona F. Sunset time and the economic effects of social jetlag: evidence from US time zone borders. J Health Econ 2019;65:210–26.

35. Fritz J, VoPham T, Wright KP, et al. A chronobiological evaluation of the acute effects of daylight saving time on traffic accident risk. Curr Biol 2020;30:729–35.

36. Malow BA, Veatch OJ, Bagai K. Are daylight saving time changes bad for the brain? JAMA Neurol 2020; 77:9–10.

37. Veatch OJ, Keenan BT, Gehrmann PR, et al. Pleiotropic genetic effects influencing sleep and neurological disorders. Lancet Neurol 2017;16:158–70.

38. Cedernaes J, Osler ME, Voisin S, et al. Acute sleep loss induce tissue-specific epigenetic and transcriptional alterations to circadian clock genes in men. J Clin Endocrinol Metab 2015;100:E1255–61.

39. Manfredini R, Fabbian F, De Giorgi A, et al. Daylight saving time transitions and circulatory deaths: data from the Veneto region of Italy. Int Emerg Med 2019;14:1185–7.

40. Linderberger LM, Ackermann H, Parzeller M. The controversial debate about daylight saving time (DST): results from a retrospective forensic autopsy study in Frankfurt/Main (Germany) over 10 years (2006-2015). Int J Legal Med 2019;133:1259–65.

41. Poteser M, Moshammer H. Daylight saving time transitions: impact on total mortality. Int J Environ Res Public Health 2020;17:1611.

42. Fabbian F, Zucchi B, De Giorgi A, et al. Chronotype, gender and general health. Chronobiol Int 2016;33: 863–82.

43. Young ME. Circadian control of cardiac metabolism: physiologic roles and pathologic implications. Methodist Debakey Cardiovasc J 2017;13:15–9.

44. Grimaldi D, Carter JR, Van Cauter E, et al. Adverse impact of sleep restriction and circadian misalignment on autonomic function in healthy young adults. Hypertension 2016;68:243–50.

45. Meier-Ewert HK, Ridker PM, Rifai N, et al. Effect of sleep loss on C-reactive protein, and inflammatory marker of cardiovascular risk. J Am Coll Cardiol 2004;43:678–83.

46. Spiegel K, Leprout R, Van Cauter E. Impact of sleep debt on metabolic and endocrine function. Lancet 1999;354:1435–9.

47. Chudow JJ, Dreyfus I, Zaremski L, et al. Changes in atrial fibrillation admission following daylight saving time transitions. Sleep Med 2020;69:155–8.

48. Elliott WJ. Circadian variation in the timing of stoke onset: a meta-analysis. Stroke 1998;29:992–6.

49. Foerch C, Korf HW, Steinmetz H, et al. Abrupt shift of the pattern of diurnal variation in stroke onset with daylight saving time transitions. Circulation 2008; 118:284–90.

50. Sipilä JO, Ruuskanen JO, Rautava P, et al. Changes in ischemic stroke occurrence following daylight saving time transitions. Sleep Med 2016;27-28:20–4.

51. Zhang H, Dahlen T, Khan A, et al. Measurable health effects associated with the daylight saving time shift. PLoS Comput Biol 2020;16:e1007927.

52. Barnes CM, Wagner DT. Changing to daylight saving time cuts into sleep and increases workplace injuries. J Appl Physiol 2009;94:1305–17.

53. Carey RN, Sarma KM. Impact of daylight saving time on road traffic collision risk: a systematic review. BMJ Open 2017;7:e014319.

54. Robb D, Barnes T. Accident rates and the impact of daylight saving time transitions. Accid Anal Prev 2018;111:193–201.

55. Coate D, Markowitz S. The effects of daylight and daylight saving time on US pedestrian fatalities and motor vehicle occupant fatalities. Accid Anal Prev 2004;36:351–7.

56. Ferguson SA, Preusser DF, Lund AK, et al. Daylight saving time and motor vehicle crashes: the reduction in pedestrian and vehicle occupant fatalities. Am J Public Health 1995;85:92–5.

57. Malhi GS, Kuiper S. Chronobiology of mood disorders. Acta Psychiatr Scand Suppl 2013;444:2–15.

58. Hansen BT, Sønderskov KM, Hagerman I, et al. Daylight savings time transitions and the incidence rate of unipolar depressive episodes. Epidemiology 2017;28:346–63.

59. Berk M, Dodd S, Hallam K, et al. Small shifts in diurnal rhythms ara associated with an increase of suicide: the effect of daylight saving. Sleep Biol Rhythms 2008;6:22–5.

60. Shapiro CM, Blake F, Fossey E, et al. Daylight saving time in psychiatric illness. J Affect Disord 1990;19: 177–81.

61. Lahti TA, Haukka J, Lönnqvist J, et al. Daylight saving time transitions and hospital treatments due to accidents and manic episodes. BMC Public Heath 2008;8:74.

62. Heboyan V, Stevens S, McCall WV. Effects of seasonality and daylight savings time on emergency department visit for mental health disorders. Am J Emerg Med 2018;37:1476–81.

63. Borisenkov MF, Tserne TA, Panev AS, et al. Seven-year survey of sleep timing in Russian children and adolescents; chronic 1-h forward transition of social clock is associated with increased social jetlag and winter pattern of mood seasonality. Biol Rhythm Res 2017;48:3–12.

64. Roenneberg T, Allebrandt KV, Merrow M, et al. Social jetlag and obesity. Curr Biol 2012;22:939–43.

65. Parsons MJ, Moffitt TE, Gregory AM, et al. Social jetlag, obesity and metabolic disorder: investigation in a cohort study. Int J Obes 2015;39:842–8.

66. Koopman ADM, Rauh SP, Van't Riet E, et al. The association between social jetlag, the metabolic

syndrome, and type 2 diabetes mellitus in the general population: the New Horn Study. J Biol Rhythms 2017;32:359–68.

67. Gaski JF, Sagarin J. Detrimental effects of daylight-saving time on SAT scores. J Neurosc Psychol Econom 2011;4:44–53.

68. Haraszti RA, Ella K, Gyöngyosi N, et al. Social jetlag negatively correlates with academic performance in undergraduates. Chronobiol Int 2014;31:603–12.

69. van der Vinne V, Zerbini G, Siersema A, et al. Timing of examinations affect school performance differently in the early and late chronotypes. J Biol Rhythms 2015;30:53–60.

70. Diaz-Morales JF, Escribano C. Social jetlag, academic achievement and cognitive performance: understanding gender/sex difference. Chronobiol Int 2015;32:822–31.

71. Wong PM, Hasler BP, Kamarck TW, et al. Social jetlag, chronotype, and cardiometabolic risk. J Clin Endocrinol Metab 2015;100:4612–20.

72. Levandovski R, Dantas G, Fernandes LC, et al. Depression scores associate with chronotype and social jetlag in a rural population. Chronobiol Int 2011;28:771–8.

73. Debyser A, Pape M, European Parliamentary Research Service. Discontinuing seasonal changes of time 2019. Available at: https://www.europarl. europa.eu/RegData/etudes/BRIE/2018/630308/ EPRS_BRI(2018)630308_EN.pdf. [Accessed 20 February 2021].

74. Dijk DJ, Vanderwalle G, Wright KP, et al. Panel discussion. Daylight saving time – forever?. 2018. Available at: https://www.sleepscience.at/wp-content/uploads/2016/10/Panel-Discussion_ESRS_ SUMMARY_final.pdf. [Accessed 28 February 2021].

75. European Biological Rhythms Society, European Sleep Research Society, Society for Research on Biological Rhythms. To the EU Commission on DST. Available at: https://esrs.eu/wp-content/uploads/ 2019/03/To_the_EU_ Commission_on_DST.pdf. [Accessed 20 February 2021].

76. Rishi MA, Ahmed O, Barrantes Perez JH, et al. Daylight saving time: an American Academy of Sleep Medicine position statement. J Clin Sleep Med 2020;16:1781–4.

77. European Commission. Commission Staff Working Document: Public Consultation on EU Summertime Arrangements, Report of Results. Available at: https://ec.europa.eu/info/law/better-regulation/ initiative/1918/publication/302607/attachment/ 090166e5bd928364_en. [Accessed 20 February 2021].

78. Blume C, Schabus M. Perspective: daylight saving time - an advocacy for balanced view and against fanning fear. Clocks Sleep 2020;2:19–25.

79. Kountouris Y, Remoundou K. About time: daylight saving time transition and individual well-being. Econ Lett 2014;122:100–3.

80. Skeldon AC, Dijk DJ. School start times and daylight saving time confuse California lawmakers. Curr Biol 2019;29:R278–9.

Sleepiness Behind the Wheel and the Implementation of European Driving Regulations

Walter T. McNicholas, MD[a,b,*]

KEYWORDS

- Sleep apnea • Driving • Accident risk • Sleepiness • Screening • Driving simulators • Treatment
- Regulations

KEY POINTS

- Sleep disturbance and sleepiness are established risk factors for driving accidents and obstructive sleep apnea (OSA) is the most prevalent medical disorder associated with excessive daytime sleepiness.
- Because effective treatment of OSA reduces accident risk, several jurisdictions have implemented regulations concerning the ability of patients with OSA to drive, unless effectively treated.
- The present review provides a practical guide for clinicians who may be requested to certify a patient with OSA as fit to drive regarding the scope of the problem, the role of questionnaires and driving simulators to evaluate sleepiness, and the benefit of treatment on accident risk.

INTRODUCTION

Disorders associated with sleepiness are recognized risk factors for road accidents[1] and obstructive sleep apnea (OSA) is the most prevalent medical disorder associated with excessive daytime sleepiness (EDS), affecting up to 1 billion subjects worldwide.[2] EDS is a key feature of OSA and EDS while driving is an important factor in motor vehicle accidents (MVA) or work-related accidents.[3] The medicolegal consequences of OSA principally relate to accident risk with its associated economic and legal consequences.[4] The risk of MVA in drivers with OSA has been quantified to range between two and seven times the risk of control populations[5] and effective therapy, usually with continuous positive airway pressure (CPAP), alleviates this increased accident risk.[6] Several jurisdictions have implemented regulations restricting the ability of patients with OSA to drive until effective treatment is demonstrated.[7] Such regulations typically include objective severity of OSA demonstrated by the measured apnea-hypopnea frequency (apnea-hypopnea index [AHI]) in a sleep study in addition to self-reported sleepiness. The importance of including both measures is emphasized by the poor association between AHI and subjective sleepiness measured by the Epworth Sleepiness Scale score (ESS),[8,9] and the continuing uncertainty about the relative importance of AHI and sleepiness in predicting accident risk.[3]

In 2014, the European Union (EU) implemented a directive that introduced regulations regarding fitness to drive in patients with OSA. This directive specifies that patients with AHI greater than or equal to 15 and associated sleepiness should not drive until effective treatment is demonstrated and physician certification is required to confirm suitability to continue driving.[10] However,

---

Author has nothing to disclose.

[a] School of Medicine, University College Dublin, Dublin, Ireland; [b] Department of Respiratory and Sleep Medicine, St. Vincent's Hospital Group, Elm Park, Dublin 4, Ireland.

* Consultants' Clinic, St Vincent's Private Hospital, Herbert Avenue, Suite 5, Dublin 4, Ireland.

E-mail address: walter.mcnicholas@ucd.ie

Sleep Med Clin 16 (2021) 533–543
https://doi.org/10.1016/j.jsmc.2021.05.003
1556-407X/21/© 2021 Elsevier Inc. All rights reserved.

considerable uncertainty prevails among clinicians about the evaluation of suitability to drive in patients with OSA,[11] which probably reflects uncertainty regarding the appropriate criteria to evaluate disease severity, particularly the evaluation of sleepiness. Although sleepiness at the wheel is a topic that extends beyond OSA, the subject of this review concentrates on driving and OSA, because this is the specific focus of the EU directive.

EPIDEMIOLOGY OF MOTOR VEHICLE ACCIDENTS IN PATIENTS WITH OBSTRUCTIVE SLEEP APNEA

OSA has been recognized for several decades to be associated with an increased risk of MVA[12] and this risk is mainly associated with the degree of EDS, which is usually subjectively assessed by the ESS.[13] In noncommercial drivers, sleepiness and OSA risk were associated with increased risk of MVA in some reports,[14,15] but not in others, especially in elderly drivers.[16–18] In commercial drivers, self-reported sleepiness was also associated with increased risk of MVA.[19–21] The estimated OSA risk was associated with sleepiness in some,[22] but not all studies.[21,23]

The average increased risk of MVA has been quantified in meta-analyses and several original reports as being around 2.5 times the accident risk of control populations[5,24–26] and a recent case control study of truck drivers reported an even higher MVA risk.[27] However, not all reports indicate an increased MVA risk relating to OSA.[28] Dose-effect relationships have been reported between OSA severity and risk of MVA in the general population.[29–32] In sleep clinic samples, the association between OSA and MVA was confirmed, although some studies found no dose-effect relationship between OSA severity and MVA risk.[26,33] Finally, some studies reported that patients with severe OSA[25,34–36] and young male patients with OSA were especially at risk of MVA.[35] However, another report from Australia found no difference in MVA occurrence between heavy-vehicle drivers with and without moderate or severe OSA.[28]

Factors Contributing to Motor Vehicle Accidents Risk in Obstructive Sleep Apnea

Reports differ on the relative importance of AHI and sleepiness as major factors in determining accident risk, which is at least partly a consequence of the poor association between subjective sleepiness and AHI.[8,9] Short sleep duration and self-reported sleepiness may also play a role.[29,37] In professional drivers, similar trends have been observed with some studies underlining a major

role for sleep deprivation,[38] sleepiness,[39] and nocturnal hypoxemia.[40] EDS has been reported as the principal factor contributing to MVA risk in some reports of patients with OSA,[41] whereas other reports found AHI to be a stronger predictor of accident risk than EDS.[42,43]

MECHANISMS AND PREDICTORS OF EXCESSIVE DAYTIME SLEEPINESS IN OBSTRUCTIVE SLEEP APNEA

Excessive sleepiness is reported as a contributing factor in 5% to 7% of MVA, and in up to 17% of accidents involving fatalities.[44] A recent meta-analysis reported that sleepiness at the wheel was associated with an increased risk for MVA with an odds ratio of 2.51.[45]

Sleepiness is a major factor contributing to the occurrence of MVAs and disorders associated with EDS are recognized risk factors.[38] A role for nocturnal hypoxemia in predicting EDS has been reported in several studies,[28,33,39] and sleep fragmentation was associated with ESS scores in some[46–48] but not in other reports.[15,49,50] Large cross-sectional population studies using more liberal definitions of EDS reported no association between EDS and sleep variables, but an association with several comorbidities,[51–53] and a strong association between subjective EDS and depression in OSA has been reported.[53–55] A genetic marker of EDS in OSA has been recently identified in the AMOT gene and the related P130 protein, but these findings need confirmation in larger datasets.[56]

Depression and obesity predicted EDS better than AHI in a large cohort of patients with OSA at diagnosis[57] and a meta-analysis found that EDS decreased after weight loss without evident relationship with changes in AHI.[58] In patients undergoing bariatric surgery, EDS was related more to metabolic variables and depression than to AHI.[59,60] A longitudinal study in the general population reported changes in EDS associated with weight gain or loss, and a significant influence of comorbidities and depression over a follow-up of 7.5 years.[61]

ROLE OF QUESTIONNAIRES AS SCREENING TOOLS FOR OBSTRUCTIVE SLEEP APNEA IN DRIVERS

The high prevalence of OSA indicates that risk stratification of high-risk populations, especially in the context of driving safety, is desirable because access to diagnostic facilities is limited. Thus, several screening questionnaires have been developed to facilitate the diagnosis of

OSA, which include ESS,[13] Berlin Questionnaire,[62] STOP,[63] and STOP-Bang.[64] These tools are easy to administer but cannot be regarded as an accurate means of assessment and thus are best used as a means of triage for identification of subjects at highest risk.

In the general population, marked variation is reported in the sensitivities and specificities for all established questionnaires (ESS sensitivity 18%–85%, specificity 22%–98%[65–67]; Berlin Questionnaire sensitivity 40%–97%, specificity 6%–100%[68]; STOP sensitivity 33%–98%, specificity 10%–95%[69]; STOP-Bang sensitivity 0%–100%, specificity 0%–100%[64,70]), even taking into account different cutoff thresholds for OSA (AHI $\geq$5, AHI $\geq$15, AHI $\geq$30). Sensitivity is highest in sleep clinic samples for all questionnaires, whereas the ESS showed an overall poor predictive value.

EVALUATION OF SLEEPINESS

Evaluation of sleepiness, especially in large populations, is difficult, and simple objective tools are not available. Furthermore, fitness to drive in this context should not be viewed as exclusively related to sleepiness and other factors, such as vigilance, may be equally important.[71] Several objective and subjective tests have been developed to assess the effects of sleep deprivation on vigilant attention and the results extrapolated to driving ability.[72]

Psychomotor Vigilance Test

The Psychomotor Vigilance Test is a 10-minute test that is easy to perform in the clinical setting.[73] Reaction times on Psychomotor Vigilance Test are similar in patients with OSA and control subjects, but patients with OSA experience a higher number of lapses and performed poorly in neurocognitive tests.[74] Psychomotor Vigilance Test may be used in the occupational assessment of professional drivers,[75] although no specific parameters have been established that could be used to predict ability to drive safely.

Maintenance of Wakefulness Test

Maintenance of Wakefulness Test (MWT) consists of four 40-minute sessions that evaluate the subject's ability to remain awake and has been demonstrated to correlate with the ability to perform on a driving simulator in patients with untreated OSA.[76–78] Subjects with short sleep latency scores on MWT (0–19 minutes) display more interline crossings and deviation from the center of the road, and subjects and control

subjects least likely to incur errors had a mean sleep latency of greater than 34 minutes.[76,79]

Oxford Sleep Resistance Test

The Oxford Sleep Resistance Test is a simpler form of MWT testing[74,80] and poor performance has been shown to be associated with previous episodes of MVA.[41] The Oxford Sleep Resistance Test seems to be a sensitive test for identifying sleepiness in patients with OSA in addition to fluctuations in vigilance, although normative data are not yet available.

Multiple Sleep Latency Test

The Multiple Sleep Latency Test is considered the gold standard for assessing sleep propensity[81] but is not designed to measure sleepiness routinely because it is time-consuming and extremely labor-intensive.[81] However, any patient with a mean sleep latency of less than 8 minutes is pathologically sleepy and this finding correlates with increased risk of MVA.[72]

Relationship Between Real Life Driving Performance and Performance on Tests of Vigilance and Sleepiness

Driving is a complex task that requires integration of psychomotor, cognitive, motor, and decision-making skills; divided attention; in addition to behavioral and emotional control. Sleepiness affects many of these factors to varying degrees, which in turn are determined by individual levels of resilience and resistance to impairment and age, gender, and baseline neurocognitive function. However, most objective tests that assess driving ability in the context of OSA are unidimensional and lack established normative data for the general population regarding sleepiness but may have value for intraindividual changes, such as before and after treatment. Furthermore, testing fitness to drive in terms of sleepiness and vigilance are unnecessary in all patients with OSA, but may have a role in a subset of drivers, such as truck drivers.[82,83]

DRIVING SIMULATORS IN THE EVALUATION OF FITNESS TO DRIVE

There is considerable heterogeneity among driving simulators, ranging from those based on a personal computer with simple graphics, using a gaming steering wheel and vehicle controls, through to fully immersive simulators involving full-size real cars that closely replicate the real driving experience. Less realistic simulators are associated with more events, in patients and normal subjects,[77] whereas more than 50% of patients with a moderate-severe OSA could complete approximately 1 hour of simulated motorway driving without deviating out of the assigned lane, crashing, and so forth.[84] Standard deviation of lane position shows the best correlation with sleepiness and performance on the simulator.[84]

Patients with OSA perform worse than normal subjects on driving simulators[85–87] and performance on simulators is worse after alcohol or sleep deprivation.[88,89] Simulated driving is worse in sleepy patients[76,78,79,90–92] across all simulator types, and females perform worse than males.[84] However, performance improves after treatment of OSA in reports that included randomized control, and case control studies.[93–95] Driving performance of sleepy individuals in a driving simulator relates only partially to real road test driving performance and simulated driving performance is unable to reliably predict real-life near misses or accidents on an individual level.[86] When comparing simulated and real driving, the strongest association is seen for driving simulation near-misses or accidents with real-life rates of near-misses or accidents, followed by the number of inappropriate line crossings and the standard deviation of lane position.

EFFECTIVENESS OF CONTINUOUS POSITIVE AIRWAY PRESSURE TREATMENT IN OBSTRUCTIVE SLEEP APNEA ON DRIVING ACCIDENT RISK

Effective treatment with nasal CPAP substantially reduces the increased accident risk associated with OSA and several reports indicate that the risk may be reduced to a level similar to the general population.[6,96] A recent report found that the risk of near miss accidents in truck drivers decreased to normal after 2 years of treatment.[97] A meta-analysis also found a significant reduction in accidents after treatment,[96] which has obvious benefits in financial and human costs.[98] In the trucking industry, CPAP-adherent patients had crash risks similar to control subjects, whereas nonadherent patients had a five-fold greater crash risk after 6 years of follow-up.[99] Many studies indicate that CPAP improves sleepiness after 1 night of treatment, although few had a randomized design.[100–103] A self-rating instrument (Sleepiness Wakefulness Inability and Fatigue Test) has been developed,[104] which improves after PAP. Sleepiness assessed by Multiple Sleep Latency Test[100] and alertness by MWT[101,105] improved after CPAP. Improvements in vigilance were found after 1 year treatment[106] and CPAP therapy was associated with objectively improved reaction times and sustained attention in drivers with OSA.[107]

EUROPEAN UNION REGULATIONS AND THEIR IMPLEMENTATION

Although the EU regulations introduced in 2014 do not distinguish between professional and nonprofessional drivers in the OSA criteria that determine driving restriction, the requirements for monitoring of professional drivers are more stringent.[10] Also, some European countries have introduced stricter regulations than those specified by the EU resulting in a large variation in legislation between different countries. The risk of MVA has long been recognized as having extra implications for long-haul truck drivers, where drowsiness while driving is common,[108] and the MVA risk is enhanced by other factors, such as alcohol consumption[42] and short sleep duration.[37,109] It is also common for patients with OSA having an accident to report a preceding history of near miss events, although the relationship with near miss MVA differs between reports.[20,110] Thus, it is appropriate to consider the history of previous MVA as part of the process of issuing or renewing a driving license.

The problem of fitness to drive in OSA has been extensively investigated in the last 30 years, but the level of evidence regarding fitness to drive remains insufficient in addition to a lack of normative data regarding most tests of vigilance or results of driving simulators. There is still a lack of simple instruments that are suitable to apply on a large scale, which could reliably indicate that a subject with OSA is fit to drive or not. Although several questionnaires have been used, their sensitivity and specificity vary according to the subjects assessed.[111]

The allocation of responsibility for driver licensing is also an important consideration. Whereas it should be the responsibility of the physician to suspect OSA and request diagnostic examination in the case of subjects renewing their driving license, the primary responsibility for issuing the driving license should remain with the relevant licensing authority. Attention should be paid to potentially important risk factors, such as a history of previous MVAs, especially where sleepiness was a likely contributing factor; the presence of obesity; or a history of snoring. Unfortunately, this is often not the case, as shown by recent surveys of physicians where considerable uncertainty regarding the necessary criteria to medically approve continued driving persists.[11,112,113] Stricter criteria for the issuing or renewal of driving licenses have been adopted in

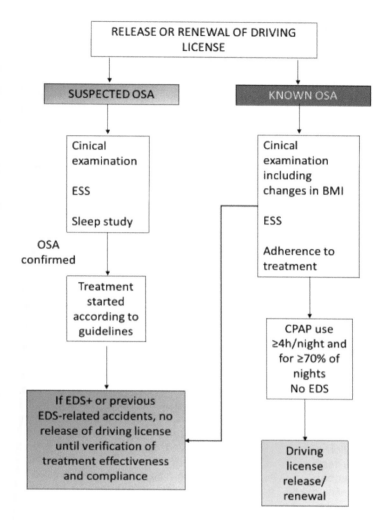

Fig. 1. The author's proposed advice on the assessment of fitness to drive in patients with OSA. This figure is an opinion and is not intended as a specific recommendation for clinical practice. BMI, body mass index. (*Reproduced from* Bonsignore MR, Randerath W, Schiza S, Verbraecken J, Elliott MW, Riha R, et al. European Respiratory Society Statement on Sleep Apnoea, Sleepiness and Driving Risk. Eur Respir J. 2020;Oct 2:2001272.)

several countries for commercial drivers, who have a higher exposure to the risk of accidents compared with noncommercial drivers because long-haul journeys and driving on divided highways are associated with greater risk than short urban journeys. A fast-track approach for sleepy drivers with OSA to allow rapid initiation of CPAP therapy has recently been tested.[114]

Although the 2014 EU directive considers OSA for the first time as a disease associated with driving risk, it remains unclear how patients with OSA should be assessed, and which factors may predict an increased driving risk. A reduced sleep latency during the MWT is used in some European countries to document increased sleepiness in patients with OSA, but the resource requirements of the test make it unsuitable to evaluate large numbers. However, only half of patients with OSA report EDS, and there is a lack of clinical markers that might help identify at-risk patients. Even in patients with OSA who are also sleepy, the prediction of MVA risk is difficult, because driver responsibility is an important factor in accident risk in such subjects, such as sleepy patients limiting their driving distances and/or stopping to rest at the earliest signs of sleepiness.[92]

In the case of CPAP-treated patients, the evaluation is more straightforward because daily CPAP compliance and efficacy are quantified by data download from the device, and there is good evidence that effective CPAP treatment greatly decreases MVA risk.[6] A recent statement from the European Respiratory Society indicated that documented use of CPAP for at least 4 hours for at least 70% of nights is enough evidence to consider a treated CPAP patient fit to drive.[115] Nonetheless, residual EDS is found in about 6% to 13% of effectively CPAP-treated patients[116,117] and the responsible mechanisms remain uncertain.[118] This aspect represents a challenge in assessing fitness to drive, although there are new drugs becoming available, such as solriamfetol[119,120] or pitolisant,[121] which may be useful in patients reporting residual EDS despite documented effective CPAP therapy and after careful attention to potential behavioral factors. A proposed management pathway for the provision of a driving license to subjects with OSA is given in **Fig. 1.**

Tests currently available demonstrate many difficulties in their practical application. For example, driving simulation represents an easy test to perform but has not yet demonstrated an ability to predict accidents in a real driving environment. Nevertheless, deviations from lane have been used to develop internal vehicle safety systems that may improve safety on the road.[122] Similarly, in-car or driver-worn real-time monitoring for drowsiness may offer some advantage in the real-time detection of subtle changes that might limit accident risk. However, care must be taken that such systems do not provide a false sense of security in a drowsy driver, who might rely on the monitoring system rather than pull over to rest when drowsy.

There is growing research interest in the identification of episodes of microsleep associated with drowsiness, which may be an important determinant of MVA risk,[123–125] and the identification of drowsiness may facilitate more applicable tests to identify drivers at risk for MVA. Another important limitation relates to the difficulty in defining vigilance, which is a complex psychological phenomenon that is different from drowsiness or sleepiness. The ESS does not measure vigilance or ability to drive, but only subjective sleepiness, and is open to manipulation by a driver wishing to minimize symptoms, especially where retention of the driving license is essential for continuing employment. Furthermore, sleepiness at the wheel may be the result of factors unrelated to OSA, especially behavioral and lifestyle factors, such as insufficient sleep duration.

CLINICS CARE POINTS

- OSA severity in the context of fitness to drive should include the objective severity demonstrated by a sleep study and the level of sleepiness, usually subjective.

- Excessive sleepiness is the most important factor relating to OSA that determines accident risk but correlates poorly with the AHI.
- If there is doubt about the validity of self-reported sleepiness, objective testing should be considered, especially in high-risk drivers.
- Effective treatment of OSA greatly reduces the accident risk and safe driving may resume once demonstrated.

REFERENCES

1. Smolensky MH, Di Milia L, Ohayon MM, et al. Sleep disorders, medical conditions, and road accident risk. Accid Anal Prev 2011;43(2):533–48.
2. Benjafield AV, Ayas NT, Eastwood PR, et al. Estimation of the global prevalence and burden of obstructive sleep apnoea: a literature-based analysis. Lancet Respir Med 2019;7(8):687–98.
3. McNicholas WT, Rodenstein D. Sleep apnoea and driving risk: the need for regulation. Eur Respir Rev 2015;24(138):602–6.
4. Krieger J, McNicholas WT, Levy P, et al. Public health and medicolegal implications of sleep apnoea. Eur Respir J 2002;20(6):1594–609.
5. Tregear S, Reston J, Schoelles K, et al. Obstructive sleep apnea and risk of motor vehicle crash: systematic review and meta-analysis. J Clin Sleep Med 2009;5(6):573–81.
6. Tregear S, Reston J, Schoelles K, et al. Continuous positive airway pressure reduces risk of motor vehicle crash among drivers with obstructive sleep apnea: systematic review and meta-analysis. Sleep 2010;33(10):1373–80.
7. McNicholas WT. Sleepiness and driving: the role of official regulation. Sleep Med Clin 2019;14(4): 491–8.
8. Deegan PC, McNicholas WT. Predictive value of clinical features for the obstructive sleep apnoea syndrome. Eur Respir J 1996;9(1):117–24.
9. Kingshott RN, Sime PJ, Engleman HM, et al. Self assessment of daytime sleepiness: patient versus partner. Thorax 1995;50(9):994–5.
10. Bonsignore MR, Randerath W, Riha R, et al. New rules on driver licensing for patients with obstructive sleep apnea: European Union Directive 2014/85/EU. J Sleep Res 2016;25(1):3–4.
11. Dwarakanath A, Twiddy M, Ghosh D, et al. Variability in clinicians' opinions regarding fitness to drive in patients with obstructive sleep apnoea syndrome (OSAS). Thorax 2015;70(5):495–7.
12. Findley LJ, Unverzagt ME, Suratt PM. Automobile accidents involving patients with obstructive sleep apnea. Am Rev Respir Dis 1988;138(2):337–40.

13. Johns MW. A new method for measuring daytime sleepiness: the Epworth sleepiness scale. Sleep 1991;14(6):540–5.

14. Quera Salva MA, Barbot F, Hartley S, et al. Sleep disorders, sleepiness, and near-miss accidents among long-distance highway drivers in the summertime. Sleep Med 2014;15(1):23–6.

15. Gonçalves M, Amici R, Lucas R, et al. Sleepiness at the wheel across Europe: a survey of 19 countries. J Sleep Res 2015;24(3):242–53.

16. Philip P, Sagaspe P, Lagarde E, et al. Sleep disorders and accidental risk in a large group of regular registered highway drivers. Sleep Med 2010; 11(10):973–9.

17. Vaz Fragoso CA, Araujo KL, Van Ness PH, et al. Prevalence of sleep disturbances in a cohort of older drivers. J Gerontol A Biol Sci Med Sci 2008; 63(7):715–23.

18. Vaz Fragoso CA, Araujo KL, Van Ness PH, et al. Sleep disturbances and adverse driving events in a predominantly male cohort of active older drivers. J Am Geriatr Soc 2010;58(10):1878–84.

19. Vennelle M, Engleman HM, Douglas NJ. Sleepiness and sleep-related accidents in commercial bus drivers. Sleep Breath 2010;14(1):39–42.

20. Catarino R, Spratley J, Catarino I, et al. Sleepiness and sleep-disordered breathing in truck drivers. Sleep Breath 2014;18(1):59–68.

21. Zwahlen D, Jackowski C, Pfaffli M. Sleepiness, driving, and motor vehicle accidents: a questionnaire-based survey. J Forensic Leg Med 2016;44:183–7.

22. Braeckman L, Verpraet R, Van Risseghem M, et al. Prevalence and correlates of poor sleep quality and daytime sleepiness in Belgian truck drivers. Chronobiol Int 2011;28(2):126–34.

23. Amra B, Dorali R, Mortazavi S, et al. Sleep apnea symptoms and accident risk factors in Persian commercial vehicle drivers. Sleep Breath 2012; 16(1):187–91.

24. Garbarino S, Pitidis A, Giustini M, et al. Motor vehicle accidents and obstructive sleep apnea syndrome: a methodology to calculate the related burden of injuries. Chronic Respir Dis 2015;12(4): 320–8.

25. Komada Y, Nishida Y, Namba K, et al. Elevated risk of motor vehicle accident for male drivers with obstructive sleep apnea syndrome in the Tokyo Metropolitan Area. Tohoku J Exp Med 2009; 219(1):11–6.

26. Mulgrew AT, Nasvadi G, Butt A, et al. Risk and severity of motor vehicle crashes in patients with obstructive sleep apnoea/hypopnoea. Thorax 2008;63(6):536–41.

27. Meuleners L, Fraser ML, Govorko MH, et al. Obstructive sleep apnea, health-related factors, and long distance heavy vehicle crashes in Western Australia: a case control study. J Clin Sleep Med 2015;11(4):413–8.

28. Stevenson MR, Elkington J, Sharwood L, et al. The role of sleepiness, sleep disorders, and the work environment on heavy-vehicle crashes in 2 Australian states. Am J Epidemiol 2014;179(5):594–601.

29. Gottlieb DJ, Ellenbogen JM, Bianchi MT, et al. Sleep deficiency and motor vehicle crash risk in the general population: a prospective cohort study. BMC Med 2018;16(1):44.

30. Shiomi T, Arita AT, Sasanabe R, et al. Falling asleep while driving and automobile accidents among patients with obstructive sleep apnea-hypopnea syndrome. Psychiatry Clin Neurosci 2002;56(3):333–4.

31. Masa JF, Rubio M, Findley LJ. Habitually sleepy drivers have a high frequency of automobile crashes associated with respiratory disorders during sleep. Am J Respir Crit Care Med 2000;162(4 Pt 1):1407–12.

32. Young T, Blustein J, Finn L, et al. Sleep-disordered breathing and motor vehicle accidents in a population-based sample of employed adults. Sleep 1997;20(8):608–13.

33. Barbe PJ, Munoz A, Findley L, et al. Automobile accidents in patients with sleep apnea syndrome. An epidemiological and mechanistic study. Am J Respir Crit Care Med 1998;158(1):18–22.

34. Arita A, Sasanabe R, Hasegawa R, et al. Risk factors for automobile accidents caused by falling asleep while driving in obstructive sleep apnea syndrome. Sleep Breath 2015;19(4):1229–34.

35. Basoglu OK, Tasbakan MS. Elevated risk of sleepiness-related motor vehicle accidents in patients with obstructive sleep apnea syndrome: a case-control study. Traffic Inj Prev 2014;15(5):470–6.

36. Horstmann S, Hess CW, Bassetti C, et al. Sleepiness-related accidents in sleep apnea patients. Sleep 2000;23(3):383–9.

37. Howard ME, Desai AV, Grunstein RR, et al. Sleepiness, sleep-disordered breathing, and accident risk factors in commercial vehicle drivers. Am J Respir Crit Care Med 2004;170(9):1014–21.

38. Carter N, Ulfberg J, Nystrom B, et al. Sleep debt, sleepiness and accidents among males in the general population and male professional drivers. Accid Anal Prev 2003;35(4):613–7.

39. Karimi M, Eder DN, Eskandari D, et al. Impaired vigilance and increased accident rate in public transport operators is associated with sleep disorders. Accid Anal Prev 2013;51:208–14.

40. Wu WT, Tsai SS, Liao HY, et al. Usefulness of overnight pulse oximeter as the sleep assessment tool to assess the 6-year risk of road traffic collision: evidence from the Taiwan Bus Driver Cohort Study. Int J Epidemiol 2017;46(1):266–77.

41. Karimi M, Hedner J, Habel H, et al. Sleep apnea-related risk of motor vehicle accidents is reduced

by continuous positive airway pressure: Swedish Traffic Accident Registry data. Sleep 2015;38(3): 341–9.

42. Terán-Santos J, Jimenez-Gomez A, Cordero-Guevara J. The association between sleep apnea and the risk of traffic accidents. N Engl J Med 1999;340(11):847–51.

43. Karimi M, Hedner J, Lombardi C, et al. Driving habits and risk factors for traffic accidents among sleep apnea patients: a European multi-centre cohort study. J Sleep Res 2014;23(6):689–99.

44. Tefft BC. Prevalence of motor vehicle crashes involving drowsy drivers, United States, 1999–2008. Accid Anal Prev 2012;45(0):180–6.

45. Bioulac S, Franchi J-AM, Arnaud M, et al. Risk of motor vehicle accidents related to sleepiness at the wheel: a systematic review and meta-analysis. Sleep 2017;40(10):zsx134–.

46. Bennett LS, Langford BA, Stradling JR, et al. Sleep fragmentation indices as predictors of daytime sleepiness and nCPAP response in obstructive sleep apnea. Am J Respir Crit Care Med 1998; 158(3):778–86.

47. Roure N, Gomez S, Mediano O, et al. Daytime sleepiness and polysomnography in obstructive sleep apnea patients. Sleep Med 2008;9(7): 727–31.

48. Seneviratne U, Puvanendran K. Excessive daytime sleepiness in obstructive sleep apnea: prevalence, severity, and predictors. Sleep Med 2004;5(4): 339–43.

49. Mediano O, Barcelo A, de la Pena M, et al. Daytime sleepiness and polysomnographic variables in sleep apnoea patients. Eur Respir J 2007;30(1):110–3.

50. Chen R, Xiong KP, Lian YX, et al. Daytime sleepiness and its determining factors in Chinese obstructive sleep apnea patients. Sleep Breath 2011;15(1):129–35.

51. Bixler EO, Vgontzas AN, Lin HM, et al. Excessive daytime sleepiness in a general population sample: the role of sleep apnea, age, obesity, diabetes, and depression. J Clin Endocrinol Metab 2005; 90(8):4510–5.

52. Kapur VK, Baldwin CM, Resnick HE, et al. Sleepiness in patients with moderate to severe sleep-disordered breathing. Sleep 2005;28(4):472–7.

53. Adams RJ, Appleton SL, Vakulin A, et al. Association of daytime sleepiness with obstructive sleep apnoea and comorbidities varies by sleepiness definition in a population cohort of men. Respirology 2016;21(7):1314–21.

54. Koutsourelakis I, Perraki E, Bonakis A, et al. Determinants of subjective sleepiness in suspected obstructive sleep apnoea. J Sleep Res 2008; 17(4):437–43.

55. Lang CJ, Appleton SL, Vakulin A, et al. Associations of undiagnosed obstructive sleep apnea

and excessive daytime sleepiness with depression: an Australian population study. J Clin Sleep Med 2017;13(4):575–82.

56. Chen YC, Chen KD, Su MC, et al. Genome-wide gene expression array identifies novel genes related to disease severity and excessive daytime sleepiness in patients with obstructive sleep apnea. PLoS One 2017;12(5):e0176575.

57. Pamidi S, Knutson KL, Ghods F, et al. Depressive symptoms and obesity as predictors of sleepiness and quality of life in patients with REM-related obstructive sleep apnea: cross-sectional analysis of a large clinical population. Sleep Med 2011; 12(9):827–31.

58. Ng WL, Stevenson CE, Wong E, et al. Does intentional weight loss improve daytime sleepiness? A systematic review and meta-analysis. Obes Rev 2017;18(4):460–75.

59. Dixon JB, Schachter LM, O'Brien PE. Polysomnography before and after weight loss in obese patients with severe sleep apnea. Int J Obes 2005; 29(9):1048–54.

60. Dixon JB, Dixon ME, Anderson ML, et al. Daytime sleepiness in the obese: not as simple as obstructive sleep apnea. Obesity 2007;15(10):2504–11.

61. Fernandez-Mendoza J, Vgontzas AN, Kritikou I, et al. Natural history of excessive daytime sleepiness: role of obesity, weight loss, depression, and sleep propensity. Sleep 2015;38(3):351–60.

62. Netzer NC, Stoohs RA, Netzer CM, et al. Using the Berlin Questionnaire to identify patients at risk for the sleep apnea syndrome. Ann Intern Med 1999; 131(7):485–91.

63. Chung F, Yegneswaran B, Liao P, et al. STOP questionnaire: a tool to screen patients for obstructive sleep apnea. Anesthesiology 2008;108(5):812–21.

64. Nagappa M, Liao P, Wong J, et al. Validation of the STOP-Bang questionnaire as a screening tool for obstructive sleep apnea among different populations: a systematic review and meta-analysis. PLoS One 2015;10(12):e0143697.

65. Sil A, Barr G. Assessment of predictive ability of Epworth scoring in screening of patients with sleep apnoea. J Laryngol Otol 2011;126(4):372–9.

66. Bhat S, Upadhyay H, DeBari VA, et al. The utility of patient-completed and partner-completed Epworth Sleepiness Scale scores in the evaluation of obstructive sleep apnea. Sleep Breath 2016; 20(4):1347–54.

67. Nishiyama T, Mizuno T, Kojima M, et al. Criterion validity of the Pittsburgh sleep quality index and Epworth sleepiness scale for the diagnosis of sleep disorders. Sleep Med 2014;15(4):422–9.

68. Senaratna CV, Perret JL, Matheson MC, et al. Validity of the Berlin questionnaire in detecting obstructive sleep apnea: a systematic review and meta-analysis. Sleep Med Rev 2017;36:116–24.

69. Chiu H-Y, Chen P-Y, Chuang L-P, et al. Diagnostic accuracy of the Berlin questionnaire, STOP-BANG, STOP, and Epworth sleepiness scale in detecting obstructive sleep apnea: a bivariate meta-analysis. Sleep Med Rev 2017;36:57–70.

70. Westlake K, Plihalova A, Pretl M, et al. Screening for obstructive sleep apnea syndrome in patients with type 2 diabetes mellitus: a prospective study on sensitivity of Berlin and STOP-Bang questionnaires. Sleep Med 2016;26:71–6.

71. Warm JS, Parasuraman R, Matthews G. Vigilance requires hard mental work and is stressful. Hum Factors 2008;50(3):433–41.

72. Gupta R, Pandi-Perumal SR, Almeneessier AS, et al. Hypersomnolence and traffic safety. Sleep Med Clin 2017;12(3):489–99.

73. Sunwoo BY, Jackson N, Maislin G, et al. Reliability of a single objective measure in assessing sleepiness. Sleep 2012;35(1):149–58.

74. Cori JM, Jackson ML, Barnes M, et al. The differential effects of regular Shift work and obstructive sleep apnea on sleepiness, mood and neurocognitive function. J Clin Sleep Med 2018;14(6):941–51.

75. Zhang C, Varvarigou V, Parks PD, et al. Psychomotor vigilance testing of professional drivers in the occupational health clinic: a potential objective screen for daytime sleepiness. J Occup Environ Med 2012;54(3):296–302.

76. Sagaspe P, Taillard J, Chaumet G, et al. Maintenance of wakefulness test as a predictor of driving performance in patients with untreated obstructive sleep apnea. Sleep 2007;30(3):327–30.

77. Mazza S, Pepin JL, Naegele B, et al. Most obstructive sleep apnoea patients exhibit vigilance and attention deficits on an extended battery of tests. Eur Respir J 2005;25(1):75–80.

78. Pizza F, Contardi S, Mondini S, et al. Daytime sleepiness and driving performance in patients with obstructive sleep apnea: comparison of the MSLT, the MWT, and a simulated driving task. Sleep 2009;32(3):382–91.

79. Philip P, Chaufton C, Taillard J, et al. Maintenance of Wakefulness Test scores and driving performance in sleep disorder patients and controls. Int J Psychophysiol 2013;89(2):195–202.

80. Bennett LS, Stradling JR, Davies RJ. A behavioural test to assess daytime sleepiness in obstructive sleep apnoea. J Sleep Res 1997;6(2):142–5.

81. Littner MR, Kushida C, Wise M, et al. Practice parameters for clinical use of the multiple sleep latency test and the maintenance of wakefulness test. Sleep 2005;28(1):113–21.

82. Aurora RN, Caffo B, Crainiceanu C, et al. Correlating subjective and objective sleepiness: revisiting the association using survival analysis. Sleep 2011;34(12):1707–14.

83. Philip P, Sagaspe P, Taillard J, et al. Maintenance of Wakefulness Test, obstructive sleep apnea syndrome, and driving risk. Ann Neurol 2008;64(4):410–6.

84. Ghosh D, Jamson SL, Baxter PD, et al. Continuous measures of driving performance on an advanced office-based driving simulator can be used to predict simulator task failure in patients with obstructive sleep apnoea syndrome. Thorax 2012;67(9):815–21.

85. Mazza S, Pepin JL, Naegele B, et al. Driving ability in sleep apnoea patients before and after CPAP treatment: evaluation on a road safety platform. Eur Respir J 2006;28(5):1020–8.

86. Risser MR, Ware JC, Freeman FG. Driving simulation with EEG monitoring in normal and obstructive sleep apnea patients. Sleep 2000;23(3):393–8.

87. George CF, Boudreau AC, Smiley A. Simulated driving performance in patients with obstructive sleep apnea. Am J Respir Crit Care Med 1996;154:175–81.

88. Hack MA, Choi SJ, Vijayapalan P, et al. Comparison of the effects of sleep deprivation, alcohol and obstructive sleep apnoea (OSA) on simulated steering performance. Respir Med 2001;95(7):594–601.

89. Vakulin A, D'Rozario A, Kim JW, et al. Quantitative sleep EEG and polysomnographic predictors of driving simulator performance in obstructive sleep apnea. Clin Neurophysiol 2016;127(2):1428–35.

90. Pizza F, Contardi S, Ferlisi M, et al. Daytime driving simulation performance and sleepiness in obstructive sleep apnoea patients. Accid Anal Prev 2008;40(2):602–9.

91. Boyle LN, Tippin J, Paul A, et al. Driver performance in the moments surrounding a microsleep. Transp Res F Traffic Psychol Behav 2008;11(2):126–36.

92. Pizza F, Contardi S, Mondini S, et al. Simulated driving performance coupled with driver behaviour can predict the risk of sleepiness-related car accidents. Thorax 2011;66(8):725–6.

93. George CF. Reduction in motor vehicle collisions following treatment of sleep apnoea with nasal CPAP. Thorax 2001;56:508–12.

94. Orth M, Duchna HW, Leidag M, et al. Driving simulator and neuropsychological [corrected] testing in OSAS before and under CPAP therapy. Eur Respir J 2005;26(5):898–903.

95. Turkington PM, Sircar M, Saralaya D, et al. Time course of changes in driving simulator performance with and without treatment in patients with sleep apnoea hypopnoea syndrome. Thorax 2004;59(1):56–9.

96. Antonopoulos CN, Sergentanis TN, Daskalopoulou SS, et al. Nasal continuous positive airway pressure (nCPAP) treatment for obstructive

sleep apnea, road traffic accidents and driving simulator performance: a meta-analysis. Sleep Med Rev 2011;15(5):301–10.

97. Garbarino S, Guglielmi O, Campus C, et al. Screening, diagnosis, and management of obstructive sleep apnea in dangerous-goods truck drivers: to be aware or not? Sleep Med 2016;25: 98–104.

98. Sassani A, Findley LJ, Kryger M, et al. Reducing motor-vehicle collisions, costs, and fatalities by treating obstructive sleep apnea syndrome. Sleep 2004;27(3):453–8.

99. Burks SV, Anderson JE, Bombyk M, et al. Nonadherence with employer-mandated sleep apnea treatment and increased risk of serious truck crashes. Sleep 2016;39(5):967–75.

100. Engleman HM, Martin SE, Deary IJ, et al. Effect of continuous positive airway pressure treatment on daytime function in sleep apnoea/hypopnoea syndrome. Lancet 1994;343(8897):572–5.

101. Hack M, Davies RJ, Mullins R, et al. Randomised prospective parallel trial of therapeutic versus subtherapeutic nasal continuous positive airway pressure on simulated steering performance in patients with obstructive sleep apnoea. Thorax 2000;55(3):224–31.

102. Hoekema A, Stegenga B, Bakker M, et al. Simulated driving in obstructive sleep apnoea-hypopnoea; effects of oral appliances and continuous positive airway pressure. Sleep Breath 2007;11(3):129–38.

103. Phillips CL, Grunstein RR, Darendeliler MA, et al. Health outcomes of continuous positive airway pressure versus oral appliance treatment for obstructive sleep apnea: a randomized controlled trial. Am J Respir Crit Care Med 2013;187(8): 879–87.

104. Sangal RB. Evaluating sleepiness-related daytime function by querying wakefulness inability and fatigue: sleepiness-Wakefulness Inability and Fatigue Test (SWIFT). J Clin Sleep Med 2012;8(6): 701–11.

105. Hakkanen H, Summala H, Partinen M, et al. Blink duration as an indicator of driver sleepiness in professional bus drivers. Sleep 1999;22(6):798–802.

106. Cassel W, Ploch T, Becker C, et al. Risk of traffic accidents in patients with sleep-disordered breathing: reduction with nasal CPAP. Eur Respir J 1996;9(12):2606–11.

107. Alakuijala A, Maasilta P, Bachour A. The Oxford sleep resistance test (OSLER) and the multiple unprepared reaction time test (MURT) detect vigilance modifications in sleep apnea patients. J Clin Sleep Med 2014;10(10):1075–82.

108. Mitler MM, Miller JC, Lipsitz JJ, et al. The sleep of long-haul truck drivers. N Engl J Med 1997; 337(11):755–62.

109. Pack AI, Maislin G, Staley B, et al. Impaired performance in commercial drivers. Am J Respir Crit Care Med 2006;174(4):446–54.

110. Ward KL, Hillman DR, James A, et al. Excessive daytime sleepiness increases the risk of motor vehicle crash in obstructive sleep apnea. J Clin Sleep Med 2013;9(10):1013–21.

111. McNicholas WT. Screening for sleep-disordered breathing: the continuing search for a reliable predictive questionnaire. Lancet Respir Med 2016; 4(9):683–5.

112. Mets MAJ, Alford C, Verster JC. Sleep specialists' opinion on sleep disorders and fitness to drive a car: the necessity of continued education. Ind Health 2012;50(6):499–508.

113. Alkharboush GA, Al Rashed FA, Saleem AH, et al. Assessment of patients' medical fitness to drive by primary care physicians: a cross-sectional study. Traffic Inj Prev 2017;18(5):488–92.

114. West SD, Downie B, Olds G, et al. A 4-week wait 'fast-track' sleep service is effective at establishing vocational drivers on continuous positive airway pressure. Clin Med 2017;17(5):401–2.

115. Bonsignore MR, Randerath W, Schiza S, et al. European Respiratory Society statement on sleep apnoea, sleepiness and driving risk. Eur Respir J 2020;57(2):2001272.

116. Pépin J-L, Viot-Blanc V, Escourrou P, et al. Prevalence of residual excessive sleepiness in CPAP-treated sleep apnoea patients: the French multicentre study. Eur Respir J 2009;33(5):1062–7.

117. Gasa M, Tamisier R, Launois SH, et al. Residual sleepiness in sleep apnea patients treated by continuous positive airway pressure. J Sleep Res 2013;22(4):389–97.

118. Vernet C, Redolfi S, Attali V, et al. Residual sleepiness in obstructive sleep apnoea: phenotype and related symptoms. Eur Respir J 2011;38(1): 98–105.

119. Malhotra A, Shapiro C, Pepin J-L, et al. Long-term study of the safety and maintenance of efficacy of solriamfetol (JZP-110) in the treatment of excessive sleepiness in participants with narcolepsy or obstructive sleep apnea. Sleep 2020;43(2):zsz220.

120. Schweitzer PK, Rosenberg R, Zammit GK, et al. Solriamfetol for excessive sleepiness in obstructive sleep apnea (TONES 3). A randomized controlled trial. Am J Respir Crit Care Med 2019;199(11): 1421–31.

121. Dauvilliers Y, Verbraecken J, Partinen M, et al. Pitolisant for daytime sleepiness in obstructive sleep apnea patients refusing CPAP: a randomized trial. Am J Respir Crit Care Med 2020;201(9):1135–45.

122. McDonald AD, Lee JD, Schwarz C, et al. A contextual and temporal algorithm for driver drowsiness detection. Accid Anal Prev 2018;113: 25–37.

123. Morrone E, D'Artavilla Lupo N, Trentin R, et al. Microsleep as a marker of sleepiness in obstructive sleep apnea patients. J Sleep Res 2020;29(2): e12882.

124. Putilov AA, Donskaya OG, Verevkin EG. Can we feel like being neither alert nor sleepy? The electroencephalographic signature of this subjective sub-state of wake state yields an accurate measure of objective sleepiness level. Int J Psychophysiol 2019;135:33–43.

125. Hertig-Godeschalk A, Skorucak J, Malafeev A, et al. Microsleep episodes in the borderland between wakefulness and sleep. Sleep 2019;43(1): zsz163.

Moving?

Make sure your subscription moves with you!

To notify us of your new address, find your **Clinics Account Number** (located on your mailing label above your name), and contact customer service at:

Email: journalscustomerservice-usa@elsevier.com

800-654-2452 (subscribers in the U.S. & Canada)
314-447-8871 (subscribers outside of the U.S. & Canada)

Fax number: 314-447-8029

Elsevier Health Sciences Division
Subscription Customer Service
3251 Riverport Lane
Maryland Heights, MO 63043

*To ensure uninterrupted delivery of your subscription, please notify us at least 4 weeks in advance of move.